# How to Build Muscle in Your Advanced Years

By Tony Xhudo/M.S., H.N.

Board Certified by

The American Association of Drugless Practitioners

# How to Build Muscle in Your Advanced Years

By Tony Xhudo/M.S., H.N.

Published by Dawn Xhudo

## Disclaimer

This information is presented to you for entertainment purposes. Neither the author or publisher assumes any liability for the information presented in this book. This book is not intended to provide any medical advice or health claims.

The purpose of this book is to provide you a compendium of information for you the reader, for entertainment purposes only. In seeking to apply any of the reference material that is presented in this book for your own purposes, please seek the advice of a medical practitioner in getting a physical examination before performing any of the exercise routines listed in this book.

## Dedication

This is dedicated to my wonderful wife "Dawn" that I love so much for being a great wife and a great mom. Without you encouraging me to write, this book would not have been possible.

I would also like to dedicate this book to all those that are approaching their "Golden Years of Life" to show them that one is never too old to begin training and accomplish what they have thought was impossible. I hope that you find my book was helpful and productive in helping you achieve the level of fitness that you've so desired.

# TABLE OF CONTENTS

1. HOW TO BUILD MUSCLE IN YOUR ADVANCED

2. PROGRESSIVE OVERLOAD-FORCING YOUR MUSCLE'S TO GROW

3. PHYSIOLOGY OF MUSCLE HYPERTROPHY & HYPERPLASIA

4. CORTISOL & IT'S IMPLICATIONS ON MUSCLE GROWTH

5. OVER TRAINING AND CORTISOL:HOW IT AFFECTS MUSCLE GROWTH

6. OVER TRAINING 101: WHAT YOU NEED TO KNOW ABOUT IT

7. WEIGHT TRAINING PRINCIPLES FOR BODYBUILDING

8. BEST EXERCISE'S FOR MUSCLE MASS

9. KEY EXERCISES: FOR MUSCLE MASS

10. METHODS TO HELP YOU MAXIMIZE YOUR MUSCLE GROWTH POTENTIAL

11. TRAINING FOR MAXIMUM SIZE

12. MAXIMIZING YOUR ANABOLIC WINDOW OF OPPORTUNITY PRE-WORKOUT/POST WORKOUT/BED TIME MEAL – PROTEIN SHAKES

13. BODYBUILDING TIPS, TRAINING, DIET, AND SUPPLEMENTS

14. YOUR BEST USE OF BODYBUILDING SUPPLEMENTS

15. MUSCLE BUILDING SUPPLEMENTS THAT INCREASE MUSCULAR GROWTH TESTOSTERONE BOOSTERS, GH-PRODUCTION, AND IGF-1 RELEASERS

16. HOW TO BEST USE PRE-WORKOUT/POST-WORKOUT SUPPLEMENTS

17. PRE-WORKOUT SUPPLEMENTS

18. POST-WORKOUT SUPPLEMENTS

19. BOOSTING YOUR HORMONES FOR MAXIMUM MUSCLE DEVELOPMENT THROUGH DIET & EXERCISES

20. BOOSTING YOUR TESTOSTERONE THROUGH DIET

21. TESTOSTERONE & GROWTH HORMONE BOOSTING SUPPLEMENTS

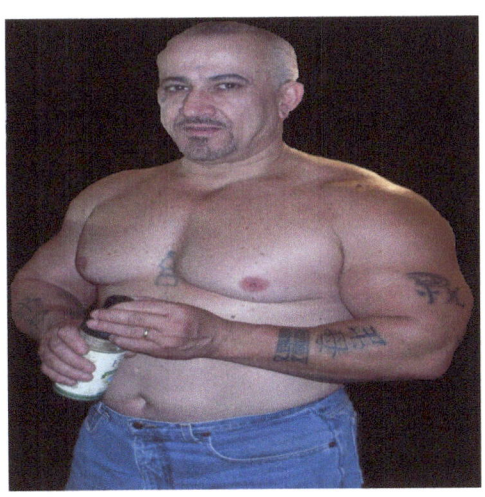

## CHAPTER 1
## <u>HOW TO BUILD MUSCLE IN YOUR ADVANCED</u>

There is no reason to believe that anyone in their old age can achieve in building a muscular body regardless if you're approaching middle age or older. It has been proven many times that muscle respond to resistance training of any kind. Getting older does not mean that we have to give up muscle strength. Your Golden years can be a time to get stronger and appear youthful as you once were, and through this book I will attempt in showing you how we can achieve a superior body that will be the envy of you're peers and associates.

With a proper diet and a planned program of resistance we can manipulate our body to a level you never thought possible. I have devoted my whole life's being on health and fitness and have proved even at my age of 55 that you can build a muscular body, as you can see by my photo on the front cover and in the book itself. But one one the greatest things about bodybuilding is that it's never too late to begin training. Recent studies have shown that you can build muscle at any advancing age as well. That's not to say that its going to be easier than it was when you were younger. Obviously with advancing age our metabolism starts to slow down along with our hormonal levels. But through diet and the correct exercise program, it has been proven that we can extend our youth a bit longer and live a healthy and vibrant lifestyle.

The human body operates on the principal use it or lose it, and those who fail to present themselves with some type of exercise stimulation will lose the ability to move as they once did. Muscle atrophy can result from failure to exercise as one gets in the older years. The body can tolerate an impressive degree of insult, such as the lack of exercise and poor diet management, up until the age 40. That's when all the mental and physical neglect begins to surface. One of the "key' aspects of maintaining physical fitness and health with the passing years is optimal nutrition. The same principle applies when your young also applies when you're middle-aged or old. You still need to get in all the required nutrients and avoid the foods that promote disease and physical degeneration.

If you are over 40 and want to build and keep your muscle, your primary focus should be on maintaining health and preventing disease that starts in the middle years of your life. That's clearly what differentiates older bodybuilders from their younger peers. At the height of their physical powers, the young often show very little concern for preventing disease or attaining some form of physical structure. All that changes when you start turning 40 or older. Even if you still choose to ignore the effects of aging, that will soon become apparent.

Good nutrition and exercise can diminish the effects of aging, or even slow down the effects associated with aging. That's why one needs to know how to eat correctly and establish some sort of healthy life style by adapting to a physical exercise program on a weekly basis. Weightlifting is one of the true ways to build muscle, whether you are young or old. Through my years of research in the health and fitness years, I've noticed a lot of the literature say that the best time to build muscle is in your 20's. However, what I have observed through my years as a professional trainer and coach, is that there are a lot of guy's in their 30's and 40's who are more muscular now than when they were younger. Obviously, we do have to consider that as one ages, our metabolism and hormonal system starts to slow down. Recuperation is another great factor that has to be considered, it stands to reason that as we get older we can't run as fast as when we were young, or recover from an all night party of alcohol and wild entertainment. But the good thing about it is, its never too late to start no matter how old we get. Men in their middle age are starting to take better care of themselves physically than they once did years ago.

I personally have been lifting weights since I was 14 years old, never knowing if I was doing the exercise correctly or not, but I loved the "muscle pump" effect that I retained after training. But eventually as the years progressed, with proper research and training, I managed to build a physique that was the envy of my peers. I also noticed that through my long years of lifting weights, I've made some of my best gains when I was in my 40's and 50's. Now at 55 years of age, I can maintain what I have very easily. Your muscles actually start to mature when your in your early 30's, that's why if you notice some bodybuilders in their later years that still compete, you'll notice that they looked much than they did when they were in their 20's.

By applying a scientific approach to training and dietary changes with the help of some supplements, you will be able to build a physique that will astonish you and you're peers. That is what this book will teach you, by addressing certain view points of training, hormone manipulation, and supplementation, you will then have all the necessary ingredients in building a muscular body. I will show you how we can build muscle in your middle age as fast as humanly possible. Lucky you that bought this book.

We will begin by paying attention to certain physiological factors of how and why muscle growth occurs with the proper training techniques and a diet designed just for muscular growth and health. There is no bull-crap about it, through all my years as an holistic practitioner and bodybuilding training I will outline a simple protocol for you to follow and have as your own bodybuilding Manuel. This protocol will work for any genetically average male providing you follow what is written. Muscle growth occurs with a progressive resistance training course. All the drop sets, giant sets, super sets, and fancy-dancy techniques of bodybuilding in the world will never be able to trump "Progress Over Load". So always try and add weight to your exercise during your workouts.

Exercise's like ___compound movements such as bench press, heavy rowing, presses, chin-ups, squats, dead-lifts, and parallel bar dips with weight___ are and have been the corner stone to building muscle as fast as possible. Done correctly, these movements have been the staple of building muscle mass from champions like Reg Park, Arnold Schwarzenegger, Dorian Yates, Ronnie Coleman, and others. Employ a sound nutritional diet with ample amount of rest days, you too can and will be able to build muscle on a week to week basis.

Sticking with the basic movements allows you to focus and put in more intensity in your workouts. A 3 day a week workout in the beginning of your program will provide sufficient amount of recovery days for you to grow. Monday-Wednesday-Friday's, 3 times a week, with 4 rest days for recovery should be fine for 3 months of training before you switch over to another routine. In the later chapters you can see sample routines that have been laid out for you. Some are based on your training level of bodybuilding, so choose one that will be appropriate to your needs.

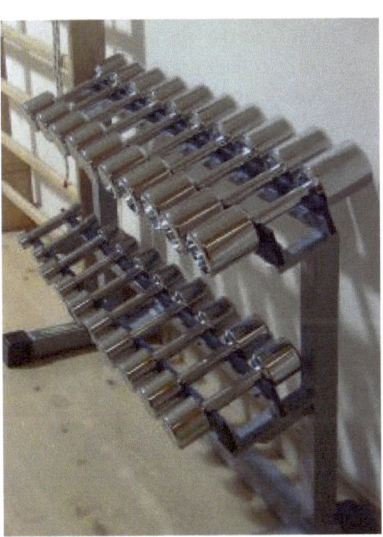

## CHAPTER 2
### Progressive Overload-Forcing Your Muscle's To Grow:

The determining factor in muscle growth is a progressive-overload of resistance training of muscle tissue. Muscle growth occurs only in a response to the stress put on the muscle. When an unusual over load *(stress)* is placed on the muscle tissue, a trauma occurs which causes small tears in the muscle fibers and the connective tissue of the muscle itself. With a sufficient break in rest and a recovery period, the body will repair these small tears with a sound nutritional plan and additional protein intake, which will add size to the muscle fibers in order to better handle the over load that was placed on it previously. This is called "Hypertrophy".

Essentially what you are doing is stressing the muscle tissue, resting and recovering, feeding the muscle for repair; hence the growth process, and then repeating the stress level over again (***progressive-overload***) forcing the muscle to grow. This is the basic philosophy in a progressive weight training regimen designed for muscle building, a gradual increase in poundage of weights one lifts will create the need for the body to make the muscles stronger and bigger. Repetitions of 3 to 6 reps have been determined to be the ideal way to go .The increase in weight loads are determined by the body as a stress response, so the genetically programmed response will be to increase muscle mass in order for the muscle to better handle the additional load placed on it. ***So, know this, muscles will only grow when they are forced to grow !***

Extra muscles will only also occur providing you feed it correctly by giving yourself the required amount of nutrients and protein.
We can't change our genetics, but we can increase our diet with a sound nutritional plan supplying the body with what it needs to put on and sustain new muscle mass through a resistance type of training we can change the demands we place on our muscles regardless of our genetic make up.

Through diet you can consistently provide the materials the body needs for additional growth of muscle to take place. The phenomenon known as the "pump" is partly a short lived example of an increased muscle cell volume, which is fluid (blood) moving into the cell of muscle tissue thereby causing it to stretch. It is this increase of cell volume that contributes to muscular growth. Research has also shown that supplements such as carbohydrates, lipids, and amino acids that increases cellular movement and blood volume within the cell causing hypertrophy to take place thus an increase in muscle size.

The cells within the muscle tissue are involved in a process called "protein turn over" which is a balanced activity of breaking down the muscles and building it back up again.

Muscles are basically built up by mainly protein and water, and because of this you have to give your body a good amount of nutritional foods. Protein is the building blocks of what we are genetically made of, and the growth of skeletal muscle mass depends on protein turn over and cellular turn over. Protein synthesis is the way the body repairs and grows muscle tissue after exercise, and is the basic component of muscle. The importance of protein intake can't be over stated and optimal protein intake based on many university studies state that it is the first step in creating an optimal environment inside your muscle cells where it can grow.

In this respect supplementing your diet with high quality protein shakes can be a big boost towards your muscular development. The human body synthesizes protein from diet at a rapid rate while the body is growing through adolescence and into adult hood. In an adult athlete , the synthesis of muscle protein is also related to how the muscles are being exercised. Muscular activity is a prerequisite of meaningful muscle development, built on protein synthesis.

During a physical workout, muscle will naturally break down , a process known as "***catabolism***", this break down includes the physical separation of muscle fibers that comprise the muscle structure. The subsequent repair of the damaged muscle is known as *"anabolism"*, which is the build up and the growth of the existing and previously damaged muscle fibers. Protein synthesis is the mechanism by which the body affects this repair and muscle growth: as a very general proposition, when the body produces more synthesized protein than it consumes through its catabolic process, muscles then will be developed.

Protein is the nutrient that attracts most attention among athletes and gym enthusiasts. After all this is perfectly logical because protein is the "key" structural component of lean muscle tissue. *In closing this chapter, if we want to get the most muscular growth possible from our protein intake, then by applying all that we have just went through in principle on muscular growth would be crucial towards your development of muscle mass gained.*

## Overview:

When it comes to muscular growth, I would like to make a point clear. In the long run when training, if the desired outcome is gains in muscle mass, you have got to become stronger and productive during your workouts. So what ever workout your doing in building muscle mass, you have to challenge yourself in making your training sessions more challenging by employing the productive over-load principle discussed earlier.

Stick with compound exercises as stated earlier, these are the exercises that will get you to experience fast muscular growth, results that you can see in no time. Never workout the same muscle group or exercise when in heavy training for two days in a row, as this will result in stalemate and over training. Your rest periods should be no more than 30 to 65 seconds between sets. Stick with repetitions in 4 to 6 range for optimal strength and 6-8 for muscle mass.

Learn to also break up your exercises every 6 to 8 weeks as to avoid stalemate and boredom. Example, if doing barbell bench press, change it to dumbbell bench press or incline bench press. Stick to and adhere to a sound nutritional diet plan providing your body with high quality protein from food sources and supplements. Understand that nutrition is more than half the battle in building muscle tissue and health. Get enough rest and sleep to recover from your heavy training sessions, and an occasional nap of 45 minutes to an hour, here or there would be of great benefit towards your muscle gains. This is when muscle growth and repair of damaged muscle cells occur.

Provide your body with ample amounts of protein every day keeping your body in a positive nitrogen state (anabolism) for muscle growth to occur and avoiding catabolism, the breakdown of muscle tissue.

Recognize the difference between fast and slow twitch muscle fibers as they correspond to muscle growth.

## Note:
The following chapters will be much more explicit and more in depth on certain topics recently discussed, such as diet and protein requirements, sports supplementation, exercising, hormonal health for building muscle mass, over training, and the little secrets muscle magazines fail to touch on.

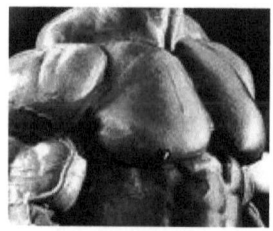

## CHAPTER 3
## PHYSIOLOGY OF MUSCLE HYPERTROPHY & HYPERPLASIA

With the belief of the inactive population concerning muscle growth , it is often led to believe that there must be a lot of agony associated with the development of muscle stimulation in your daily workouts, but not so !
In effect resistance training recruits more muscle fibers and thus causing your muscle's to grow stronger and bigger from your weight training. The science behind muscle building and growth is a complex biological process that involves certain biological steps. The good thing is that one really does not need to know everything about muscle hypertrophy and attain a Ph.D in the process, but all you really need to know is some basic steps that will help you build some serious muscle. You may ask, so how do muscle's grow ?

Well, let's find out in a more simplified way that will lead to a better understanding in allowing you to accomplish this. As your training in the gym with resistance exercise's, hypertrophy begins to take place. Muscle hypertrophy is an increase in the size of the muscle through an increase in the size of its component cells. Hyperplasia is the splitting of muscle fibers that results in a greater number of muscle fibers the same size as the originals.

Most theories are based on the idea that lifting weights or resistance training breaks down the muscle cells, and growth of the muscle results from the over-compensation in order to protect the body from future stress. The human body breaks down and rebuilds all of the muscles every 15 to 30 days, and rebuilding the muscle peaks 24 to 36 hours after training that can continue at an increased rate for as much as 72 hrs. there after. Muscles also are composed of 2 basic type of fibers, slow twitch and fast twitch muscle fibers. ***Slow twitch muscle fibers*** are those that are used in primarily endurance type of activities, such as long distance running, and weight resistance training with high repetitions of light weights will help to stimulate and develop these types of muscle fibers. Note that also training these types of muscle fibers (slow twitch) will not result in any gain of muscle mass. Just look at the world class long distance runners and see how lanky and  thin these runners are.

***Fast twitch muscle fibers*** are capable of a greater force that tire easily and have the least endurance than slow twitch muscle fibers. Fast twitch muscle fibers are those used in an explosive force as such activities like sprinting or power lifting. Weight resistance type of training with heavy weights will help to develop fast twitch fibers and potentially help you produce significant gains in muscle mass. Just think of the world class sprinters  with those thick muscular legs.

So to build muscle and gain weight fast you must focus on the fast twitch muscle fibers during your training sessions and emphasize this important factor in your training regime.

This means that one must focus on training for strength and not endurance on any given workout day. Training with heavy weights and low repetitions, and not with light weight and high repetitions. Also bare in mind that genetics do play an important part that determines the proportions of slow twitch muscle fibers to fast twitch muscle fibers that a person's muscle's contain. There are those individuals that contain a higher percentage of fast twitch fibers that will gain muscle mass relatively more than those with a high percentage of slow twitch muscle fibers, and they a called "Hard Gainer's". But that does not necessarily mean that those born with a high percentage of slow twitch fibers can't gain muscle mass just as easily as those born with fast twitch muscle fibers. Through a progressive weight lifting resistance course, any hard gainer can make expect to see the same results as those gifted good genetics, and that is what this whole book is about. We're going to make that happen for you!

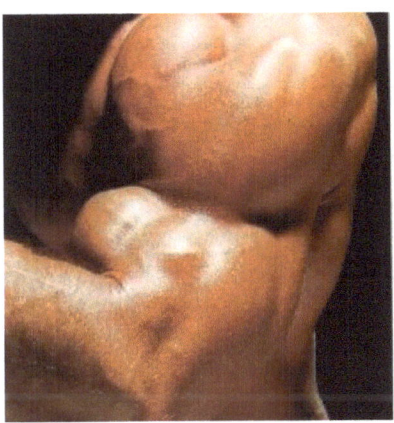

## CHAPTER4
## CORTISOL & IT'S IMPLICATIONS ON MUSCLE GROWTH

Cortisol, is a bodybuilders worst nightmare for muscle-building. Cortisol is termed catabolic as it has the opposite effect to testosterone, insulin and growth hormone (GH) in that it breaks down muscle tissue. Cortisol is released by the adrenal glands in response to mental and physical stress. It is also the body's primary catabolic hormone. It is therefore essential that levels of cortisol do not go in excess, as otherwise it can lead you to a muscle building halt. It is the excess levels that concern us that is problem for bodybuilders, not cortisol itself. However, your body does require cortisol to maintain important processes during prolonged periods of stress. Without cortisol, you would go into shock and die if exposed to severe trauma. But for some reason our own bodies just don't know when to quit producing it when agitated or stimulated. Excess levels that are not under control can cause a range of health problems which are:

➤ **Reduce the output of GH and testosterone.**

- ⊼ **Reduce muscle tissue and cause abdominal fat.**
- ⊼ **Can cause an imbalance of blood sugar levels.**
- ⊼ **Impair memory and learning**
- ⊼ **Impair immunity levels.**
- ⊼ **Can cause disease's such as Cushing's Syndrome.**

Although cortisol release can't be prevented, it can be controlled through dietary means and with supplementation. Cortisol is at it's highest during the morning hours in preparing the body for on-coming day, and it is also at it's lowest during night time when we are sleeping. Certain beverages that have caffeine are soda's, coffee, and the super high energy drinks that they sell commercially. One study showed that individuals with too much cortisol found it impossible to lose weight even with the perfect diet and exercise program. Another important factor to consider is over training and spending pro-longed hours in the gym. This can only negate all the hard work spent in the gym trying to build muscle.

So by having excess levels of cortisol, an athlete is at a great disadvantage in trying to successfully build muscle tissue. As for weight training the more the intense the exercises are, the higher the release of cortisol will be. But The more experienced athletes or bodybuilders are in training often show little or no change in cortisol output. Because they have adapted, some by intensifying their workouts to an hour or less. University studies done on weightlifting and athletes showed cortisol release to be at it's highest at one hour of weightlifting resistance training. Some signs of excess cortisol production in the body are; water retention, excess fat in the central area of the body like the stomach and buttocks, and the failure to increase in muscle growth and strength. Cortisol also promotes the release of "myostatin", a protein that breaks down muscle tissue.

Signs of inadequate levels of cortisol are weakness and fatigue. Cortisol also has an inverse relationship with testosterone, growth hormone, and insulin. When cortisol levels are high, it depresses the effects of these other anabolic hormones.

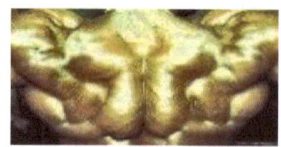

## CHAPTER 5
## OVER TRAINING AND CORTISOL:HOW IT AFFECTS MUSCLE GROWTH

This is a topic that is so common in the bodybuilding, which so many young beginners fail to understand and apply. The spend hours, upon hours, as a beginner in gym's throughout wondering why they aren't gaining any muscle mass or growth. As an experienced bodybuilder myself with over 40 years of experience, i have also as a beginner failed to understand and apply myself when I first began training.

You then you begin to wonder whats going on here ? I'm taking the same supplements as what every one else is taking but still no growth? Yet we search muscle mag's back in the day looking for certain training routines that our favorite champions are doing,failing to comprehend that they got that way by some other means that we're not aware of or their not saying.

We begin to think that maybe their doing some special routine done in a certain way. So we try and emulate what they are doing, two to four exercises per body part,five to six sets of each exercise ,and now where in the gym for 2 hours trying to finish our special routine of the champions, and still no muscle mass?

By the time i realized that i was way over training myself thinking that more is better, and in reality less is better when it comes to muscular growth. As i soon discovered this concept and changed a few things in my training sessions, I finally began to make some head way, WOW ! did that make all that happen? i spent less time in the gym about 45 minutes to an hour at most, and lowered my sets and exercises per body part,and then boy did my gains accelerate !

As you go along in this chapter i will explain to you this very important concept of muscle development in detail. So here we go to new muscular growth!

### Cortisol Overview:

To increase muscle mass you need to adhere to, that all aspects of bodybuilding and lifestyle are completely balanced. That means you are consuming a proper diet pertaining to your particular needs as a bodybuilder,your also doing just enough training

for that particular muscle group,time allotted that's spent during your training session.

All these factors play a big part in developing your muscular growth. The most import factor to consider that can hinder muscular growth is cortisol. You have to realize also that just about any type of intense training can bring on the release of cortisol, and athletes with the highest levels of cortisol are bodybuilders, due to their over training sessions.

Cortisol is triggered by  a stress response, it can be through a mental type of stress or physical. Your body does not know the difference. Considered a catabolic hormone, meaning it eats muscle tissue and can stop you from making any positive muscle gains, But yet its still a necessary and vital hormone that we need to survive.

Cortisol can't also be totally eliminated from the body, as it is needed to maintain important processes during prolonged bouts of stress. But as it pertains to bodybuilding, cortisol will reduce the body's ability to process amino acids and build muscle.

Excess levels of cortisol will also inhibit growth hormone levels by stimulating the release of growth hormone antagnostics.  As powerful as cortisol is, there are ways to control it for our particular needs in bodybuilding. The ***first step*** is to make sure we get enough sleep each day,because a lack of sleep is basically a signal to the body that there is some form of stress going on here.

The ***second step*** is to not over train during each of your workout sessions. More is not necessarily better. But that doesn't mean to not put enough intensity in your workouts either,because muscle is torn down while we workout,but grows when we rest up.

***Third,*** eliminate certain un-necessary trigger points that activated cortisol, like too much caffeine in your daily diet, coffee, soda's, and lifestyle.

***Fourth,*** introduce supplements that help with balancing cortisol levels.

### Supplements That Help To Control Cortisol Levels

*Vitamin - C* – a study done in the 90's showed that weightlifters taking extra Vitamin - C boosted their cortisol to testosterone ratio by 20%.

*Vitamin B5 & B2* – needed by the adrenal glands to manufacture adrenal hormones that helps to balance cortisol levels.

*Phosphatidyserine* – 300 mgs two times per day lowered cortisol levels by 15-30%.

*Cissus Quadrangularis* – studies done on this herb lowered cortisol levels by 32%.

*Rhodiola Rosea* – a great adaptogen that helps to keep stress levels under control and calms the mind.

*Magnolia Bark* – an effective herb that is used to control anxiety and stress which therefore helps lower cortisol.

*Royal Jelly* – very high in vitamin B5 that is specific in producing adrenal stress hormones.

*DHEA* – a natural hormone of the adrenal glands that declines after the age 30 seems to have some powerful anti-cortisol effects.

*L-Glutamine* – the most abundant amino acid in the muscle tissue that research suggests that glutamine levels may be a good indicator of over training. Glutamine directly prevents the cortisol induced degradation of muscle tissue wasting.

*Siberian Ginseng* – used extensively by Russian and Asian athletes to combat cortisol levels prior to training.

*Ashwaganda* – a powerful adaptogen used for stress control and the over-production of cortisol.

*Horny Goat Weed* – studies have shown that this herb enhances stamina and reduces cortisol produced as a result to post exertion exercises.

*Notes: Try and keep workouts under 1 hour and train efficiently and intensely, studies do show that cortisol levels rise and peak after 1 hour of intense training.*

*Spike your insulin levels after your workouts by consuming high glycemic carbohydrates that will help lower post induced high cortisol levels after training. Since insulin interferes with cortisol and it may enhance cortisol removal from the blood stream.*

One other thing that we have to be concerned with is over training during your workouts. We have to keep in mind that as we age our recuperative abilities are not what they were when you were young, so we have to be as diligent and efficient as we can be. That is another "key" component that we have to keep in mind as we're working out. So, with the information given to you about cortisol, we now have a good understanding of how cortisol can ruin our chances of gaining muscle quickly. Over training goes hand in hand with cortisol. By keeping your workouts under one hour and taking the proper supplements to help keeping cortisol under control, we can now minimize its effect on our capability to gain muscle rapidly. You'll thank me in the end when its all said and done.

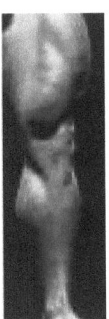

## CHAPTER 6

### OVER TRAINING 101: WHAT YOU NEED TO KNOW ABOUT IT

How does one know that their over training? When some people train 5 to 6 days a week and perform 6 to 10 sets on full body workouts,that's over training. You have to realize that there are so many training programs out there and so many of them contradict one another its ridiculous,and its know wonder that so many beginners over train.

*We have where you can do a whole body session in one workout.*

*2 to 3 day split routines.*

*4 day split routines.*

*5 day split routines.*

*Volume training,etc.,etc.*

I'm sure you get the picture,but basically over training is where you train your body above its capacity and it can't recover and adapt quickly enough for your next training session. Which means that you're training too hard with not enough rest and recuperation.

### Symptoms of Over-Training:Overview

With me through the years of being a personal trainer & coach, I've noticed the symptoms quite easily. For one, when you see the same individual day in and day out training in the gym along side of you through the weeks and months, and they basically look the same. You kind of know that something is wrong here ? Also the big factor for me was they would be at the gym before me and still be there trying to finish up their workouts,and in the mean while I'm done and hitting the showers already, you get the picture?

### But here are the most common symptoms of over training;

*You just can't seem to get any bigger after weeks and months of training.*

*Your energy levels die out in the middle of workouts.*

*Your muscles are always sore the next day following your workouts.*

*You have a general lack of energy that seems to never go away.*

*You're sleeping habits are off ,and never quite feel that you slept enough.*

*You just don't seem to get motivated for your next workouts.*

Seems obvious doesn't? if you have any of these symptoms then your over training and failing to make the gains that you need to make and look the way you want to.

If you're training correctly you should feel energized and always looking forward to your next workout day. You should always also be making steady and consistent gains on a monthly basis. That right there should make one realize that something is wrong with your training.

Your workouts should always feel progressive and positive on a weekly basis as well. If your diet is correct and you're getting enough of the protein your body requires, you're supplementing your workouts with the proper supplements and sleeping correctly. Then you should be able to make all the gains you need providing all of the above.

Often at times, over training can happen to the best of us,even experienced bodybuilders go through it. If that's the case it always best to just shut it down and take a week or two off and just regroup allowing your body a complete recovery period. I myself will apply this practice, because at times we as experienced bodybuilders fail to realize that after say six to ten months of training, we forget to take a break of a week to two weeks off. Some this can be a great thing as it just brings on new growth once you start again with your training.

That's always a good idea,taking breaks after so many months of working out. It sort of brings a new sense of enthusiasm to the table. Taking two week breaks gives your muscles a break and yourself a chance to re-evaluate your progress thus far,and to either modify or change certain things of your     training or diet, supplements, etc.

I have always made great progress when I started to take rest periods of a week or so and often noticed just by doing that I've gotten bigger in size. Now that's a good thing when that happens, isn't it?

So in reality,the best person to design your muscle building routine is you ! With of course some help with what I've given you here in this book !

### Over Training Syndrome: How to Avoid it

Over training occurs when athletes train far and above their recovery process not allowing the body to recuperate properly. This is a common practice with so many novice and well advanced athletes thinking that more is necessarily better. Which is not the case, as too much overload and or too little recovery just leads to training regimen's that can backfire and lead to no progress at all in regards to muscle growth. Bodybuilding and weightlifting requires a balance between over load and recovery, and here in this chapter we will deal with how to avoid over training syndrome the proper way.

While there are many proposed ways to objectively test for over training , the most accurate  and sensitive way are measurements in your psychological demeanor, symptoms and signs as your change of mental state, decreased positive feelings in your sport,fatigue,depression and failure to make bodybuilding progress which usually appears after a few days of intense training. Here are some of the most common symptoms to help you better distinguish over training syndrome.

### Over Training Signs and Symptoms On The Nervous System

1. Early onset of fatigue during training.
2. Weak appetite.
3. Trouble sleeping
4. Irritability.
5. Depression.
6. Weight loss.
7. Increased metabolic rate.

## Over Training Effects on Hormone Levels

1. Decreased levels of testosterone.
2. Decreased Thyroid hormone levels.
3. Increased levels of Cortisol.

The increased levels of cortisol along with decreased levels of testosterone are a deadly combination as this leads to muscle tissue breakdown, which will ultimately lead to muscle loss. There are many studies that have indicated the body's hormonal response in regards to over training affects the whole body and that it can have a serious affect in your muscle building process.

The best treatment for over training is simply to just rest ! How much rest you need depends on on how long you've been in this cycle, but generally sometimes its just better to take a week or two off from training and allow for a complete recovery. Use the time off to go over your training routine and see where you may have done too many exercises per certain body parts, reevaluate where you may have over done it. Take additional nutritional supplements that may help you in sustaining your energy level and give your recovery process a jolt that will help prevent future cycles of over training. Supplements like **"Glutathione"** can help prevent over training tremendously by strengthening your immune system. The amino acid **Glutamine** can combat the various stresses brought on by heavy training.

Supplementing with Glutamine has been shown to keep the body in a positive nitrogen balance as well as combat excess cortisol which is a big plus. Given Glutamine's low cost availability, it would be of great benefit to include this amino acid in your training program. Glutamine can be a great anabolic aid in that it prevents excess cortisol and muscle wasting syndrome. I generally take 10 to 30 grams of Glutamine myself and can honestly say it has helped me a great deal.

You may also want to look into some herbal cortisol inhibitors like **Ashwaganda, Schizandria, Rhodeola Rosea, and Phosphitadyserine**. Cortisol is catabolic to muscle tissue and excess levels will hinder your muscle building efforts to a stand still. These supplements will help keep your cortisol levels down allowing you a wide open path to muscle growth.

### Overview Solutions in Combating Over Training Syndrome

1. Take a break from training to allow time for recovery.
2. Reevaluate your training program, by reducing the volume of exercises and time

spent in the gym.

**3.**     Make sure you're getting enough sleep and rest for adequate recuperation.

**4.**     Massage the affected muscles, and take a cold to hot shower to stimulate hormonal release.

**5.**     Ensure that your caloric intake and protein matches that of your expenditure during training sessions.

**6.**     Address your training with supplementation designed to combat excess stress placed on muscles during intense exercise's. Utilizing supplements listed above.

**7.**     Learn to change your weightlifting programs around never doing the same movements for months at a time to prevent boredom.

**8.**     Shock your muscles with different training principles, as muscle can get complacent if doing the same type of routine over and over again.

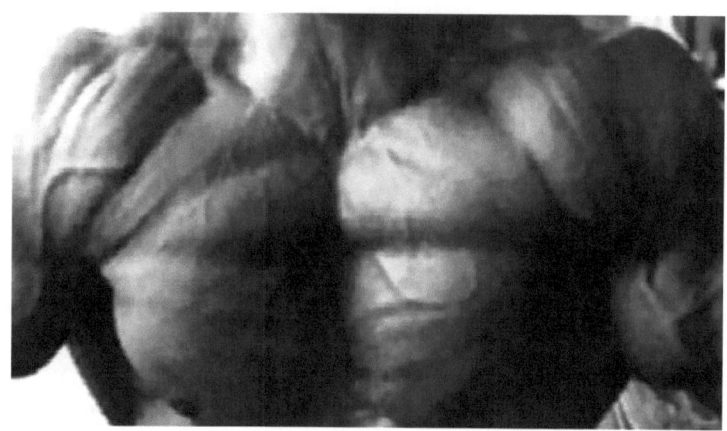

## CHAPTER 7
## <u>WEIGHT TRAINING PRINCIPLES FOR BODYBUILDING</u>

Without a constant change in your training regimen, the body will absolutely go stale. The likely reason ? You haven't thrown anything new into the mix. Muscles need to be shocked, challenged or lets say waken up, because just like anything else, it will eventually get boring and then we wonder why we're not making any muscle gains. Progression is the key to new muscle growth, and we do have the blue-print for you here in this chapter.

The Weider principles is a list of weightlifting truisms gather and honed by the father of bodybuilding "Joe Weider" that have stood the test of time through the years past. There are 24 of these principles, and it is highly recommended that you look into these principles to learn and advance your muscle building efforts.

**Muscle Priority Training** – this is working out the most weak or particular body part that needs more emphasis on building up.

**Progressive Overload** – in making additional muscle gains you need to work harder in a progressive manner from one workout to the next trying to increase the weight in each session, doing more reps,sets, or decrease your rest periods between sets.

**Pyramid Training** – is incorporating a range of lighter to heavier weights for each exercises. Starting out light with higher reps of (12-14) to warm-up the muscle, then gradually increase the weight in each successive set while lowering your reps (6 to 8). You can also reverse this procedure by moving - from high weight and low reps to low weight and high reps, aka reverse pyramiding.

**Instinctive Training** – is experimenting to developing an instinct as to what works best for you by using your training results along with past experiences to fine tune your program. Go by feeling in the gym, if you don't feel like doing biceps because you feel they may have not recovered enough from the last workout, then do another body part instead.

**Flushing Training Technique** – is training one body part with multiple exercises (3-4) before you train another. The "flushing" is your sending a maximum amount of blood and nutrients to that particular area of the muscle to stimulate growth.

**Isolation Training** – this technique allows you to work an individual muscle without involving adjacent muscles or muscle groups. A press down for triceps rather than close grip bench press is an example of an isolation movement.

**Cycle Training** – devoting portions of your training to specific goals for strength,mass or getting cut. This can help decrease your chance of injury and add a variety to your routine. Cycle periods of high intensity training and low intensity to allow for recovery and create new gains.

**Elective Training** – incorporating a diverse set of variables, such as sets, reps and exercise schemes into your workout. Body part should utilize both mass-building multi-joint moves and single joint exercises.

**Continuous Tension** – this is done by not allowing a given muscle to rest at the top or bottom of the movement by controlling both the positive and negative portions of a rep and avoiding momentum to maintain constant tension throughout the entire range of motion.

**Peak Contraction** – squeeze your contracted muscle isometrically at the end point of a rep to intensify effort. Hold the weight in the fully contracted position for up to two seconds at the top of an exercise.

**Super Set Principle** – performing sets of two exercises for the same or different muscle groups back to back with no rest period in between.

**Tri-Set Principle** – is done by performing three consecutive exercises for a particular muscle non-stop without resting.

**Giant Sets** – this is done by performing four particular exercises for a one muscle group performed in back to back fashion without rest in between.

**Burns** – continuing a set past the point at which you can lift the weight through a full or partial range of motion with a series of rapid partial reps. Do this as long as your muscles can still move the weight, even if its only for a few inches.

**Cheating Principle** – using a momentum (a slight sling of the weight) to overcome a sticking point as you fatigue near the end of a set. While doing barbell curls, for example, you might be able to perform only eight strict reps to failure. A subtle swing of the weight or a slightly faster rep speed may help you get 1 to 2 additional reps. Cheating principle is normally used for advanced bodybuilders.

**Forced Reps** – have a training partner assist you with the reps near the end of a set to help you train past the point of momentary muscular failure as your training partner assists you in the lift of the movement. Example, when performing a maximum set of reps, say 6 to 8, he will then help with a slight lift getting past 6-8 reps, say to 10 reps with his help.

**Negative Training Principle** – resist the downward motion of a heavy weight. For example, on the bench press, use a weight that's 15% to 25% heavier than you can typically handle, and fight the resistance on the way down of the movement. Then have your training partner assist you on the positive portion of the rep helping you on the way up of the exercise.

**Partial Reps** – do reps involving only a partial range --- at the top, in the middle or at the bottom --- of the movement.

**Pre-Exhaustion Principle** – pre-exhaust a muscle with a single-joint exercise before performing a multi-joint movement. In leg training, you can start with leg extensions (which target the quads) before starting a set of squats (which also work the glutes and hamstrings).

**Rest – Pause Principle** – take brief rest periods during a set of a given exercise to squeeze more reps out of a set by using a weight that you can lift for 2-3 reps, rest as long as 20 seconds, then try another 2-3 reps. Take another brief rest and go again for as many reps you can handle, and repeat one more time.

**Descending or Drop Sets** – after completing your reps in a heavy set, quickly strip an equal amount of weight from each side of the bar or select lighter dumbbells. Continue to do reps until you fail, then strip more weight off to complete more reps.

**Iso-Tension Principle** – between sets (or even between workouts), flex and hold various muscles for 6-8 seconds, keeping them fully contracted before releasing. Competitive bodybuilders use this technique usually to enhance their posing ability through increased muscle control.

There you have it ! Over 20 weightlifting principles to help guide you through your bodybuilding goals. These principles have guided many athletes through the years on their way to stardom, or personal endeavors.
With regards to your training, you will be actually using some of these principles in the exercise program for muscle mass in the following Chapter of "Mass Gaining Exercises".

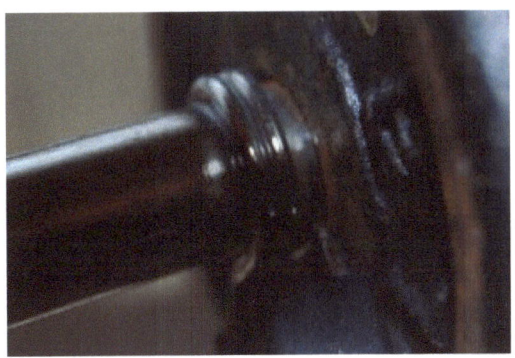

## CHAPTER 8
## BEST EXERCISE'S FOR MUSCLE MASS

There are many exercises that will basically build muscle mass, but we are going to actually list those that many bodybuilders rely on for muscle mass. The best way to do that is by specific movements as mentioned in the begging of the first chapter. These specific exercises target the large muscle groups of the body. These exercises for maximum muscle growth that are considered the best, have been accounted for years ago. They have and will always be the number one exercises for the single purpose of how to gain weight fast, and nothing compares to that, and they will never be bested. Basic or compound exercises allow you to lift more weight, and the more weight you lift, the bigger you will become.

With that in mind, what are the compound exercises which are the ones that are the best for maximum muscle mass? Compound lifts, or multi-joint lifts, are weightlifting exercises that force you to use more muscle groups, preferably 3 or more. For example, the bench press is a compound exercise, although the primary muscle used is the chest muscles, your shoulder,triceps are also helping you lift the weight.
The tricep push downs, however, are an isolation movement or single-joint exercise that basically isolates the triceps, and triceps only, a single muscle. Since this exercise just isolates a single muscle, your triceps, it doesn't involve or stimulate nearly as much muscle growth as compound lifts would do.
Although they are many other different compound movements, you must focus on only those that stimulate the most amount of muscle and allow you to lift the heaviest weight possible.

Here are the best compound exercises or mass building exercises that you must include in your training regimen if you expect to build maximum muscle mass in the shortest amount of time. This is the main focus of this book, building maximum muscle mass in the shortest amount of time. If you follow this program and apply what you've learned by reading this book, you will then not be disappointed, I assure you !

If your workouts do not include any of these compound movements, well then don't expect to grow. Ask any serious bodybuilder in the gym and they will tell you that compound exercises is a sure fire way to build muscle mass fast. One of the greatest advantage of compound exercises is you can do a whole body workout in just a few exercises in just a few minutes. And in contrast to isolation exercises which usually focuses on only a single muscle group, compound exercises allows you to limit your isolation exercise sets for instance because you've already worked your muscle groups to a certain extent.

There is over 100 years of evidence that these compound exercises actually work faster, because compound movements stress the largest amount of muscle groups the quickest.

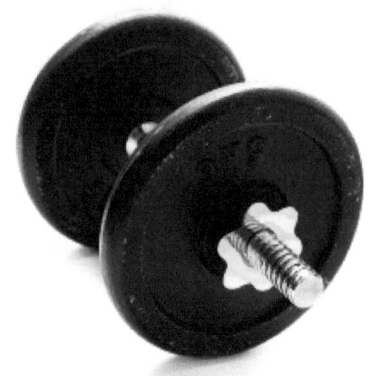

## CHAPTER 9
## KEY EXERCISES: FOR MUSCLE MASS

Here are the grandaddy of all muscle mass compound exercises that you must include in your training regimen if you expect to build muscle mass in the least amount of time.

1. **Barbell bench press** – (targets -chest muscles, shoulders and triceps)
2. **Squats,barbell** - (targets the whole leg muscles, quads, hamstrings, and calves)
3. **Barbell rowing** – (back muscles, lats-upper and lower, rear delts, and biceps)
4. **Pull-ups** – (back muscles, biceps, rear deltoids)
5. **Military press** – (shoulders, front deltoids & medial deltoid, triceps, traps)
6. **Dead lifts** – (leg muscles, lower back, biceps, forearms)
7. **Parallel Bar Dips** – (complete chest muscles, triceps, and shoulders)
8. **Power Cleans** – (forearms, back, legs, traps, biceps, shoulders)
9. **Clean & Jerk** – (forearms, biceps, triceps, shoulders, traps,legs)

Try starting some of these of exercises by adding lets say, an example routine would be like this – a whole body workout. Beginning with a warm up of course, light cardio (treadmill 10 minutes). **Workouts will be 3 days a week – Monday-Wednesday-Friday's, Rest days are Tuesday,Thursday, Saturday and Sunday (rest days are most important)**

### Beginner's Weightlifting Routine

1.  *Squats* – 2-3 sets of 10-12 reps
2.  **Bench Press** – 2—3 sets of 6-8 reps
3.  **Dips** – 2-3 sets of 8-10 reps
4.  ***Pull-ups*- (same as above)
5.  **Dumbell** rowing-(same)
6.  ***Miltary press*** -(same)
7.  **Upright Rowing**-(same)
8.  **Barbell curls**-(same)
9.  Close grip tricep press downs - (same)
10. **Abs** 2 sets of however many you can do)

As you can see in the sample routine above we have listed 5 of the compound exercises along with some isolation movements. Two to three months of this say, sample routine would be an ideal type of workout that literally targets muscles from head to toe. Emphasis should always be on a progressive light increase in weight, especially on the compound movement exercises. Try not to be sloppy but always perform your exercises as strictly as possible. The only weight lifting principle that will be employed here would be the progressive-overload principle. This is how you're going to build your muscle mass as quickly as possible.

You can of course vary your sets and reps as you go along and get comfortable with what you're trying to do. Most importantly try and not to exceed, to be in the gym for over an hour, 45 minutes to one hour maximum is allowed, anything after that will be counter productive and will only lead you to over training syndrome. Use the clock as your intensity booster keeping an eye out for your time allotted for your workouts.

**Intensity** and **progression** are **two key important factors** to consider along with the gate keeper, the clock!

This is what builds your muscles efficiently and gets you the results that you would want to see in no time,trust me and you will be very happy with the results. I have never met anyone that's utilized this system and managed to gain any muscle mass, not in over 30 years of training.

### Sample Exercise Routine For The Advanced Athlete;also done 3 days a week

**Warm-ups – light cardio, treadmill or cycling. (10 to 15 minutes)**
1.  **Squats** – 3 sets x 10-14 reps (compound exercise)
2.  **Leg Extensions**- 2-3 x 8-10 reps
3.  **Bench Press** – 3 sets x 4-6-8 reps (compound exercise)
4.  **Dips (with weight strapped on waist) – 3 sets x 6-8-10 reps (compound exercise)**
5.  **Barbell rowing – 3 sets x 4-6 reps (compound exercise)**
6.  **Power Cleans -  3 sets x 3-5 reps**
7.  **Military press- 3 sets x 5-7-8 reps (compound exercise)**
8.  **Dumbell laterals** – 2-3 sets x -6-8 reps
9.  **Barbell curls**- 2-3 sets x 6-8 reps
10. **Dumbell preacher curls** – 2-3 sets x 6-8 reps
11. **Abs**

As you can see above on the advanced training routine that all the ***compound movements are all done in 3 to 4 sets and are high lighted.*** Based on your particular energy level it would be hard for me to gauge your endurance, so this basically the start off point. You may be able to do more ? That's determined by you, as I often do not like to count sets, I tend to use the "Instinctive Training Principle" and just train according to how i'm feeling on that particular workout day. My reps are actually done the same way,i go by how I feel. My main focus in training is to never train more than one hour for any given training day, and rely on intensity and progressive overload principle. This type of training has never let me down in gaining as much muscle mass as I ever needed, nor for anyone else for that matter.

## 4 days a Week Split Training Routine For the more Advanced Bodybuilder

### Example  Workout

#### Monday – Chest/Back
#### Chest-Exercises
1.      Barbell Bench Press- (note compound movement)
2.      Dumbell Fly's
3.      Pullovers

#### Back Exercises
1)      **Barbell Rowing (note compound movement)**
2)      Cable machine Rowing
3)      Wide Grip Cable Pull downs Behind Neck
4)      Close Grip Thumbs Apart Cable Pull downs

*Note: Sets and repetitions are not listed but can be generally 2-3 sets of each exercise and the repetition range can be anywhere from 6 to 8 reps. Rest periods should be kept to a minimum as stated earlier keep an eye out on the all important time keeper of opportunity 45 minutes to one hour maximum time.*

**Important Fact:** University studies have revealed that cortisol (the catabolic hormone) is secreted the most after 45 minutes to an hour of training, so with this you need to keep it mind to maximize your muscle building efforts  always when training. That is why I stress this particular fact many times during the writing of his book, **I just can't stress this  enough.**

#### Tuesdays – Legs/Calves

#### Leg – Exercises

1.      Barbell Squats – (compound movement)
2.      Leg Press Machine-
3.      Leg Extensions -
4.      Calf Raises with weight on shoulders-

#### Wednesdays

Rest

### Thursday – Shoulders & Triceps

1) Military Press – (compound movement)
2) Upright rowing
3) Dumbbell side laterals
4) Tricep Close Grip Press-
5) One Arm Dumbell Tricep Extension

### Friday – Legs & Biceps

1. Squats
2. Leg presses
3. Calf raises
4. Barbell cheat curls
5. Preacher curls
6. Incline dumbbell curls

### Saturday & Sunday
Rest days

*Note: All sets are generally 3-4 and reps 6-8 range.*
*You have to remember, that muscles grow in capacity to the over-load placed on them, providing of course your diet plan is intact to feed the growth of new muscle, you will not go wrong but be amazed of how quickly you can put muscle mass on. It's a week to week growth in my book if everything is done correctly !*

Those of you that's willing to work hard on just a few compound exercises can also expect results like this as well. Even hard gainers will do excellent on compound movements. The problem sometimes with hard gainers is that their to busy employing routines of the champion bodybuilders and not including any of these exercises but instead focusing on special isolation exercises instead. Isolation exercises are fine to do, and there is basically nothing wrong in doing them. They do provide growth, but what we are after is muscle growth that will come as quickly as possible.

Now that you know the key muscle building mass exercises for maximum growth in record time, I want you to use them to your advantage. If you haven't tried any of them before, your in for a treat. They are tough to do, well some of them are, like the clean & jerk, power cleans and squats literally take everything you've got, but the results are very gratifying once your muscle are bulging with new growth!

So just work hard at it and imply what you've learned here, eat lots of good food, use the section on nutrition and get plenty of rest, then just get ready later on to buy some new shirts and pants, because your old one's will no longer fit you.

I myself have spent my whole life studying nutrition, health, and fitness. Through the years as a personal trainer I have had the pleasure of helping those that were hard gainers in changing their whole outlook on this type of training, and by employing certain key points, they have transformed themselves into a muscle making machine that has gotten them to where they never thought was possible before. Like I said in the beginning of this book, muscle building isn't rocket science, its basically like a simple math formula, that by just adding a few key exercises, knowing how your muscles grow, and understanding what they need for growth, lots of quality foods, proteins, essential fats, complex carbs, all fit into the equation of rapid muscle growth!

## Sample Training Systems

There are so many training variations now, that it's no wonder beginner's in weightlifting never make any gains. There are 3 days a week whole body training, with 4 days of rest; Four days a week split training with 3 days of rest in between. Two times a day, double split training sessions, am and pm, working different body parts on different occasions and days. We will break down each of these different ways and of how you can best use them to your advantage. Most of the top professional bodybuilders around the world train in these advanced ways of working out the particular body parts, emphasizing muscle growth even further. But these guys are pro's and they've been at it for quite sometime now and make a good living at it as well.

**Below is a list of the current different type of training systems you can use.**

**3 Days a week whole body workouts** – (generally used for beginners, but advanced lifters can use this as well) great for bulking up muscle-mass.

**4 days split system** working out different body parts on different days splitting the upper body one day and the lower body the other day-(allows one to put in extra effort to particular muscle groups) used more so with advanced lifters. **Example – day 1 chest/back, day 2 thighs/hamstrings & calves, day 3 shoulders/calves, day 4 biceps/triceps/abs.**

*Note: Because this workout splits the body up in over 4 days, you can do more sets per muscle group. This split system is better suited for advanced bodybuilders, and frequency wise 4 days is good for that hard muscular look with minimum fat. And it is the hard gainers that sometimes benefit most by 4 day a week training doing 2 days on and 1 day off, 2 days on and 2 days off.*

**2 times a day split system am and pm workouts**- (focuses more-on particular body part specialization & isolation) used by advanced bodybuilders for competition.

**3 Day Split Training** – In this the whole body is worked out in a period of three days, Example -day 1 / chest/back/abs ; day 2 thighs/hamstrings/and calves. Day 3 shoulders/triceps/biceps.

**Push/Pull Workout System** – This involves utilizing all pushing exercises one day- like , bench press, military press, etc. and then all pulling type of exercises the next day, such as rowing, cable pull downs, curls, etc. (Popular method used)

**One Body Part Per day Split** – This involves training only one body part per day until you have completed the whole body cycle for the week. Example – one day you work on chest, the next day legs,and the following day shoulders,etc,etc. This type of routine works out well for some people and not for others. It basically allows you to really emphasize single body parts and blow through the intensity barrier.

**The Antagonistic Muscle Workout** - Training the apposing muscles like,back and chest together on the same day of workout. The idea here is to provide maximum blood flow to the entire torso area for muscle growth. Or like training the biceps and triceps together, same reason as before.

Well as you can see there are many different types of systems that you can use in the world of bodybuilding, and probably at one point in another you most definitely will use, as I have in my 35 years of working out. I just wanted you get a grasp on the different methods used for different ways of new muscle growth.

I know your probably thinking, well, which one is the best one to use ?  To answer that question, lets say the best one to use is the new one that you have started. Meaning that muscles need to be shocked or challenged as I have mentioned earlier. They grow when new techniques are applied, again of course you eat well and consuming the right amount of necessary nutrients.

Always try to keep the muscles guessing, so they do not become complacent or stale. That is another important factor to consider and remember. That's why some bodybuilders do very well in gaining muscular growth, and yes genetics do come into play here, but in general do understand what I'm trying to tell you ? Its not very complicated. You will see for yourself once you've really understood the concepts that I have laid out for you in this book. Keep this book by your side and make notes when you can, keep a log of your training progress as you also go along, as this way you will be better able to gauge your muscle growth on a weekly basis, yes I said weekly basis ! That is how quickly you can make your muscles grow. You don't have to wait 6 months to a year for your buddies to notice, you can achieve a very good muscular physique that quickly.

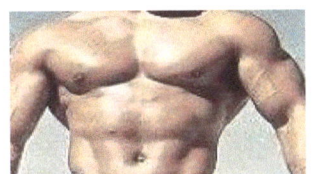

## CHAPTER 10
## METHODS TO HELP YOU MAXIMIZE YOUR MUSCLE GROWTH POTENTIAL

Consistency is the key to success in maximize your potential in bodybuilding. In this segment of the chapter I'm going to maximize your success by giving you certain key points you would want to add to your bodybuilding venture. Little tricks that you can do in and out of the gym to extend your muscle growth capabilities. For some individuals, you may have already followed this or have applied it before, and for those that have not, you will then benefit by it and have learned something new. The more of these steps you follow, the faster you will build your body.

1)      **Always stretch** after you've completed your training sessions. I know your probably thinking,shouldn't I stretch before I lift ? The answer is No!

The reason you don't stretch before you lift weights is , you don't want to injure yourself, as this will make you more susceptible to injury. Stretching before workouts when the body and muscles are cold  is a huge mistake. By stretching after your workouts when your muscles are already warm and flow of blood supply and nutrients, you'll be activating more muscle fibers that help create new muscle cells. These new muscle cells also play an important role in the recovery process.

2)      Always try and employ at least **two or more compound movements** in every training sessions, as they target  and recruit more muscle groups to your advantage. The other benefits to compound lifts are; growth hormone production, increased production of testosterone, and activation of smaller muscle groups.

3)      **Utilizing proper muscle building diet** for your body type. This would be in my opinion as I have stated on many occasions in this book as thee most important factor. As hard training requires quality protein,fats,and carbs in order for muscle growth to occur.

4)      **Always take advantage of that anabolic window** – post workout meals, and unfortunately there are only a few of these anabolic windows of opportunity to put your body in this anabolic state. But by not taking the advantage of this window of opportunity you will put your body in the opposite state "catabolism". Which is the state where your body is sacrificing muscle tissue instead of muscle growth. Your goal is to try and stay in this anabolic mode as much as your body allows you to.

**Anabolic Windows:**

**Phase 1** – comes 15 minutes following an intense workout and you have 45 minutes to an hour to capitalize. With a high protein meal.

**Growth Phase** – Takes place 1 to 2 hours following phase 1.

**Recovery Phase** – Takes affect following 2 hours after the growth phase.

**Your Secret Anabolic Window** ? Is bedtime meal or protein shake, this is one of those crucial windows for most of your muscle growth to occur. By providing your body with the proper amount of high quality food necessary for optimal muscle growth. (see chapter on diet).

5)      **Keep a log** of everything you do during your workouts, exercises, sets, reps, record of weight used for each exercise, foods you eat, etc.

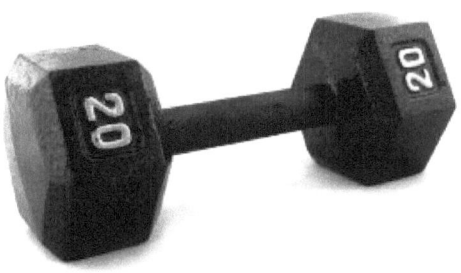

## CHAPTER 11
## TRAINING FOR MAXIMUM SIZE

When training for muscle size you have to remember that everyone is different and everyone responds differently to different training methods, however when it comes to maximum muscle size everyone will respond to a progressive over-load principle. Its just natural for muscles to grow when a heavy load is placed on them, muscle cells will split and grow new muscle cells to accommodate the load placed on it.
Give some of these mass techniques a try to kick start your muscles if you have reached a plateau.

1)    **Training for size:** Reps are 4 to 8 range. Anything lower than that is good for strength, and when a weightlifter trains for 1-3 reps they are getting their tendons, ligaments and central nervous systems stronger, however you are not really causing any muscle hypertrophy in the 1 to 3 rep range. So what is the best solution to cause muscle hypertrophy ? The 4-8 repetition range stimulates muscles instead of ligaments and tendons. Which means the 4 to 8 rep range is the best method to cause muscle cell growth.

**2) How to Get Huge Leg Muscles** – One of the best ways to cause your leg muscles to grow fast is by doing deep full heavy squats for reps of 20 being the maximum weight you can handle. Example – lets say that you can squat 300lbs for 15 reps, next time try to do 300lbs for 20 reps. This will cause amazing growth to your legs as as well as stimulating upper body growth too.

3)    **High Intensity Training -(HIT)** Is doing an exercise to an all out single set to failure. This is also known as "High Intensity Training" (HIT) means to lift weights for only two days a week, and performing two exercises only. What you are doing is, trying to do two all out exercises for the most intense sets of your life. Such as, if your bench is a 405lbs max for 1 repetition , instead reduce the weight to down like 225lbs and take 5 seconds to bring it down to your chest  and then go up slowly with it for a set of  12 reps to failure. By training this way and doing heavy negative overload principle for reps can also help you attain growth.

Always remember to rest and recover  properly as this type of training can really tear down muscle tissue, take also lots of supplements to support your muscle growth, because the bottom line is, if you do not recuperate correctly then you will tear down muscle tissue and they will never get a chance to heal and growth.

## Example of High Intensity Training (HIT)

### Day One

1)      **Squats – 315 x 20 reps, then you do a 1 rep max of 350lbs**
2)      **Deadlifts – 315 x 20, then you do a 1 rep max 405lbs.**

### Day Two

1)      **Bench Press – 255 x 8, 350lbs x 1 rep max.**
2)      **Military Press – 185 x 6-8 reps, 225 1 rep max.**
3)      **Bent Over Rowing – 225 x 6-8 reps, 275 x 1 rep max.**

*Note: Don't forget your post workout meal with a protein shake to follow.*

4)      **Stretching** - stretch after every muscle group is finished working out. This will help to improve muscle recovery that much quicker allowing for maximum blood flow to muscle cell tissue.

5)      **Progressive Over-load –** The most important aspect of muscle growth is to overload the muscle with heavy weight more than what you are accustomed to, or decrease your rest periods in between sets.

6)      **Do Power Lifting Exercise's –** for a short while, 4 weeks of this type of training will shock your muscles into new growth.
**(Example)**

1)      **Full Squats -**
2)      **Bench Press -**
3)      **Power Cleans-**
4)      **Clean & Jerk -**
5)      **Dead Lifts -**
6)      **Dumbell Curls-**
7)      **Close Grip Tricep Press-**

**This routine you can do *3 days a week*, working out the whole body. Mind set should be heavy weights with *low reps of 3 to 6 , and 1 rep max* at the end of each last set per exercise.**

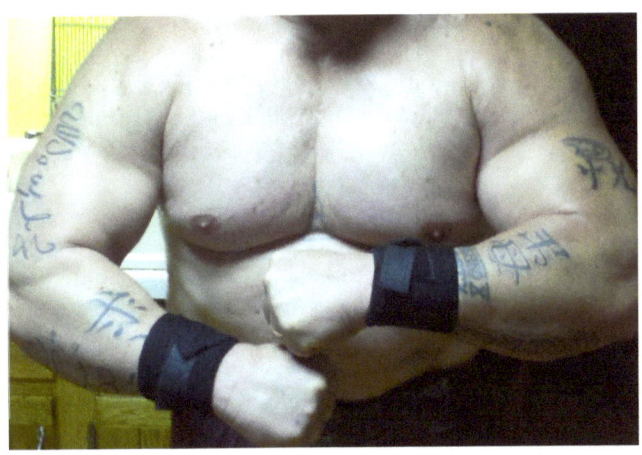

## CHAPTER 12
### <u>Maximizing Your Anabolic Window Of Opportunity</u>
### <u>Pre-Workout/Post-Workout/Bed Time Meal – Protein Shakes</u>

There are opportune times when it is crucial to feed your muscle for optimal growth. These are the critical windows of anabolic opportunity that must be adhered to and maximized for your benefit. If your diet is stable and geared for muscle building efforts, these three windows of anabolic activity will be the ones that stimulate growth and provides you with a golden opportunity for muscle building.

*Your pre-workout meal* can be a *light protein/carb mix, (liquid shake) with 15 to 25 grams of protein, and 30 to 45 grams of complex carbohydrates* taken 1 to 2 hours before your workout session allow enough time for digestion to take place.
*Your post workout meal* should consist of a protein shake of *40 to 50 grams of whey protein*, and *2 table spoons of Flax seed oil;* after you finished your training, consume your high protein shake of *whey protein isolates or whey hydrolyzed protein* for its rapid absorption in the digestive tract. *Your post workout meal is considered the most important meal of the day,* with the *second being your protein shake before bedtime*. The basic goal of proper post-workout and pre-workout nutrition is to quickly and efficiently provide your muscles with a high quality meal of amino acids, complex carbs,and essential fats. To rebuild what you have broken down and to allow for new growth, muscle hypertrophy.

Studies have repeatedly shown that time(anabolic window) is truly of the essence, the sooner the body is provided with nutrition the quicker it will exist from its catabolic state and enter in its anabolic mode, the less muscle you will lose and the quicker you will start to build new muscle. A recent 12 week study says that those who failed to consume a post workout meal or protein shake immediately after training suffered a lower metabolism, loss of fat free mass, and had clear indications of muscle loss – while those who did consume a post workout meal/shake significantly gained a increase in lean muscle mass.

With post workout meals or protein shakes you actually would want a faster digesting carbohydrate mix to elicit an insulin response, which surges nutrients and glycogen back into your muscles for repair and growth. Another important aspect to keep in mind is with post workout meals, you would want almost all carbs and protein with just a little fat in the mix as too much fat will slow the absorption of the glycemic response which is not what you would want.

## Carbohydrate To Protein Ratio's

Research suggests that studies done on this subject show that a ratio of 2:1 carbs to protein seems to be the ideal combination to maximize muscle cell repair and boost the metabolism for long term fat loss.

**Pre-Workout/Post-Workout Ultimate Protein Shake Formula's**

### Pre-Workout Protein/Carb Shake

*12 to 15 ozs of skim milk or water*
*15-20 grams of whey protein isolate's or hydrolyzed*
*30 to 45 grams of carbs*
*10 grams of glutamine powder*
*5-10 BCAA's*
*5 grams of creating monohydrate*
*10 grams of colostrum (bonus) great for a natural IGF-1 response*
*papaya enzyme or bromelian*

### Post-Workout Protein/Carb/EFA's Shake
*12 to 15 grams of skim milk*
*35 to 45 grams of whey protein hydrolysates*
*2 tablespoons of flax seed oil*
*5 grams of creating mono hydrate*
*10 grams glutamine*
*5-10 grams BCAA's*

### Bed Time Muscle Building Formula
*12-15 oz's of skim milk*
*35 grams of micellar casein protein*
*10 grams of glutamine*
*10 grams of colostrum*
*papaya/bromelian enzymes*
*10 grams of colostrum (bonus additive) igf-1 response*

**Note:** *This is the combination that I have been using myself and have been recommending to my clients that works very well, and the results are astonishing. On workout days I would consume 3 protein shakes a day along with my regular meals of breakfast,lunch, and dinner. On non-workout days I would consume my protein shakes 2 times a day being breakfast and bedtime. You can also just stay on the 3 protein shakes a day Monday thru Friday, skipping the weekends to give your digestive system a break.*

*These protein shake formulas listed are super charged with everything you need to maximize your growth potential.*

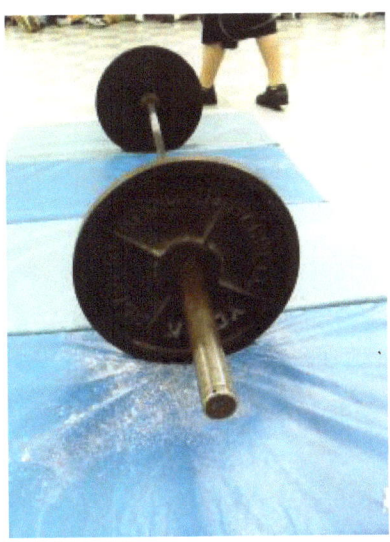

## CHAPTER 13
## <u>BODYBUILDING TIPS, TRAINING, DIET, AND SUPPLEMENTS</u>

This chapter will basically summarize some of the important facts to consider and help you to remember key points made throughout the previous chapters.

**1.**    As a general bodybuilding rule, always make it a habit to do more compound exercises than isolation exercises. It is the compound exercises that build the majority of muscle tissue, and should always be performed first at the start of your workouts while your fresh and rested.

**2.**    When training for muscle mass,always try and increase the work load by making the weight heavy as you can for the recommended repetitions of 4 to 6 reps.

**3.**    Big Movements build big muscles, like bench press,squats, dead lifts, military press, rowing ,pull ups, and dips. Think of these as the exercise staple.

**4.**    Building muscle, also involves stretching after every exercise performed. Stretching the muscle at the bottom of the movement and at squeezing the muscles it at the top.

**5.**    Barbell Squats is a must, you have to perform this exercise, because squating is the biggest muscle building exercise there is. Its not so much for the legs, but also stimulates upper body growth as well. Squating involves so many muscles and is so taxing on the body that it forces the body to release growth hormone (GH). Which basically affects all muscle growth of the body, not just the legs. Was also considered "Arnold Schwarzenegger's" favorite exercise of all.

6.      Always try and aim for improving certain aspects of your training workout from the previous week before. It can be extra reps, sets, more weight, etc.

7.      Don't over train, more is not necessarily better, meaning more time spent in the gym. Go by how your body feels, you should be leaving the gym feeling as though you could do more. If you don't feel that way, but feel tired by the end of your workout. Then that is a sign that you've done too much! Re-evaluate you're training program and see where you're doing too much of certain body parts.

8.      Keeping a train log of your workouts can become like your training partner, make sure you log the amount of weights used to keep better track of your progress. Make notes of certain points that you've noticed. Keep track of what is working for you and what isn't working.

9.      Prioritize your training to bring up certain lagging body parts, make them your main focus on what needs improving.

10.     Plan your workouts ahead, knowing what you're going to do before you walk into the gym. Thinking about what you what to achieve.

11.     Most important, be consistent in your scheduled wokouts, try not to miss any workouts. Remember you only get out of it, what you put into it, so don't miss any workouts !

12.     Learn your diet, when you start your muscle building diet plan, you need to learn everything about the food you are going to be eating. How many calories,carbs,proteins,and fats in every food group. The more you learn about your food, the easier it will be to plan your diet for muscle growth and fat loss.

13.     Treat your meals like fuel for your body.

14.     Keep well hydrated, make sure you're drinking enough fluids (3 liters). **Remember dehydration inhibits muscle growth, and can cause muscle wasting syndrome**.

15.     Make sure you're getting a balanced intake of essential fatty acids,omega3's, omega 6, and omega 9. Look for a product called Udo' Choice, perfect supplement!

16.     In trying to gain muscle mass, make sure you eat every 2-3 hours.

17.     Your carbohydrate intake should be of complex carbs, (except with your post-workout meal/shake) to provide you with long lasting energy levels.

18.     Supplement your diet with a good multi-mineral, anti-oxidants, and glutathione for your immune system. Will help with the recovery process.

**19.**     Use dextrose in your protein shakes, dextrose is the simplest of simple carbs and it can give you the best possible insulin spike, which nothing else compares.

**20.**     If you are over 35, it's not a bad idea to supplement your diet with a testosterone boosters. As this is the average age testosterone starts to wind down.

**21.**     If you have a skinny build, it would be a good idea to use a weight gaining supplement. They do give you a huge boost in calories, along with the essential nutrients like protein, carbs, and essential fats. Good brand weight gainer's are "Optimum Nutrition's-Serious Mass Gainer", and "BSN's - True Mass" both are equally as good, but I like the taste of "BSN's" products.

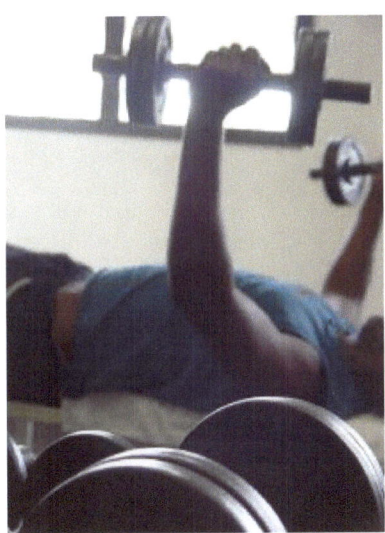

## CHAPTER 14
## YOUR BEST USE OF BODYBUILDING SUPPLEMENTS

If your goal is to gain muscle mass and establish overall health, then your best bet is to consider choosing whole foods first and supplements second. Whole foods can create and provide almost the same health response as some supplements can. Their called supplements for a reason, and that's to supplement our daily diet with nutrients that we can't get from certain foods.

So based on what you're trying to establish health wise, and muscle building, you should then plan on creating a sound diet that will compliment your body with the raw materials it needs to build muscle and a training program that will encourage muscle growth. You build muscle through diet and training. By just taking supplements alone devoid of food will only lead to poor health and all kinds of health problem. Bodybuilders in the past have always created incredible physiques without supplements back in the day. They only had whole quality foods at their disposal, which worked for them on building muscle.

But that's not to say that all supplements are bad, of course not. I'm a big supplement user myself and can attest to their effectiveness. In today's market of sports nutrition, supplements have advanced so fast, that compared to when they first came out with your basic B-complex vitamins, vitamin and minerals,vitamin E, Vit-C, etc..

Today we have herb's, Pro-Hormones, Dhea, amino acids, BCAA's,CoQ10, Acetyl-L-Carnitine, Creatine in many forms, high quality proteins -Hydrolyzed, Isolates, Micronized Glutamine, Alpha Lipoic Acid, and the list goes on and on. With the supplements we have at our disposal today, they can be used very effectively in establishing faster muscle gains to suit our particular needs.

They can also open the door for those who can't seem to maintain a solid diet and gain any muscle. The best muscle enhancing supplements, used correctly, can also give the body much more muscle building power when combined with the right foods. While whole foods are superior to supplements, supplements are vastly superior to not getting the nutrition you need. Without the proper muscle building nutrition, your muscles simply will not grow.

When it comes to building muscle, there are a few that will suit our purpose in enhancing our muscle building capabilities. I will list those according to what they do and how to use them to your advantage.

## Weight Gaining Supplements

1.      **Meal Replacement Powders** – offers you the capability to actually drink your meal in a high calorie, protein, carbohydrate, and essential fatty acid formula fortified with all the necessary nutrients your body needs to gain muscular weight quickly. Can also be used with your regular meal intake for extra protein and calorie-rich shake. Good brand names are *Met-Rx,Pro-Labs,BSN,Optimum Nutrition,and Labrada Nutrition.*

2.      **Whey Proteins** – high quality protein formula used to provide the body with extra necessary protein to build muscle, which includes all of the whey proteins, isolates, hydrolysates, and concentrates. Brand names that are good - *Optimum Nutrition, MHP, BSN, and Dymatize.*

3.      **Creatine Monohydrate** – helps the body to workout harder and longer resulting inmore muscle gains. Creatine has also been shown to help with protein synthesis as well.

4.      **Essential Fatty Acids** – you get these from products like fish oil capsules, flax seed oil, borage oil, and evening primrose oil. Fatty acids are essential to build muscle and helps the body to produce more testosterone, plus serves to control estrogen conversion from too much testosterone. *Udo's choice is a good one to take.*

5.      **Glutamine** – helps reduce and prevent exercise induced stress,protein synthesis,muscle glycogen,and helps also in preventing muscle wasting syndrome. Take at least 20 to 30 grams of glutamine daily that will provide a favorable anabolic environment for muscle anabolism.

**6.** **Weight Gain Powders** – loaded with high calories, protein, essential fatty acids, and vitamins and minerals. Also used to fortify a weight gaining diet by supplementing extra necessary nutrients for quick weight gains. Good brands to follow are *BSN-True Mass, Optimum Nutrition – Serious Mass, and MHP's – Up Your Mass.*

**7)** **Protein Bars** – great way to get extra protein in between meals. Some protein bars have high calories.

**8)** **Bee Pollen Granules** – a very good all around natural vitamin,mineral,amino acids, and enzyme supplement to take, loaded with valuable nutrition. Take with your protein shake or meal replacement, can also be taken before workouts for sustained energy levels.

**9)** **Waxy Maze** – a fast digesting carbohydrate that will help cause a rapid insulin spike necessary for anabolism to take place. It can be added to your protein powders, weight gain formula as well for extra carbohydrates and calories. Considered one of the best forms of carbohydrates thats easy on the digestive system.

**10)** **Water** – keeping the body hydrated well is crucial to muscle development ,as dehydration can, and will cause muscle wasting syndrome. Drink at least 3 liters of water daily

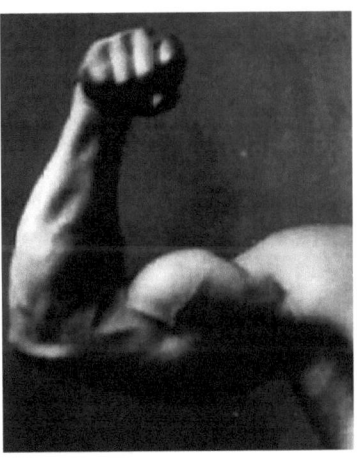

## CHAPTER 15
### MUSCLE BUILDING SUPPLEMENTS THAT INCREASE MUSCULAR GROWTH TESTOSTERONE BOOSTERS, GH-PRODUCTION, AND IGF-1 RELEASERS

**Royal Jelly** – I bet you didn't expect to find this natural product here, did you ?
This natural product from nature's busiest workers, is an all around product that helps your body combat stress induced exercise's, helps the body make testosterone, provides natural amino acids, vitamins, minerals, enzymes, and very high in vitamin B5, a natural

cortisol suppressor, and is actually used by many health enthusiasts as an anti-aging supplement. Considered a nutritional power house! *But when purchasing make sure its kept cold or it will spoil.*

**Mucuna Prureins** – A herbal testosterone releaser, GH stimulant, that is often used in the sports supplement market as an ergogenic aid in many testosterone and Gh fomula's. High in natural L-dopa, in which it is typically extracted for those with Parkinson's Disease. Mucuna helps to boost your (GH) production and testosterone that can provide benefits in muscle recovery and growth.

**Alpha-GPC** – increases the ability of the pituitary gland to produce GH to act on cells to produce muscle growth. Often used with mucuna prureins in Gh stimulating formula's.

**Creatine Monohydrate** – found in high amounts in red meats, creating has become a main stay product in the supplement world. Helping the body with energy production (ATP) and muscle cell dysplasia, can also be taken with your protein shakes to provide more of a muscle building kick.

**Cordyceps Extract** – used in traditional Chinese medicine for treating circulatory disorders and respiratory problems, cordyceps actually has amazing health benefits that will help you build muscle by also stimulating testosterone production as well. When buying, make sure it's the extract and that its standardized for 40% or higher of polysaccharides to get maximum benefits from it. Is also becoming very popular among athletes for its endurance related attributes. I myself have used cordyceps and can attest to its recuperative capabilities and energy level in the gym.

**Mooyimo Extract (mumie)** – mooyimo is an exotic, effective, and until recently a secret enhancement product from the mountains of Russia. Mooyimo has been used by Russian athletes in the Olympics for decades. Rich in bioavailable fulvic, humic, and mineralized organic acids, thus making it the ultimate Adaptogen. Mooyimo has restorative and anabolic effects, including the activation of the anabolic process in different organs and systems (blood, liver, muscles, lymphatic system, central and peripheral nervous systems, skin, hair, and the gastrointestinal tract). Mumie has become extremely popular with Russian and Eastern athletes allowing them them to train during periods of high intensity training and in recovery. Mumie can also be an effective at preventing age related-hormonal disorders, and so, it should be strongly considered as a nutrient for non-competitive athletes who participates in fitness programs. Mumie comes in as a highly recommended product for use by serious athletes and anyone else that participates in strenuous activities. Short term cycles of mumie is all that is needed by one looking to try the product, two weeks on one week off allows it to perform to its maximum level.

**Colostrum** – considered the first milk of human and animal life. Colostrum is a nutient rich pre-milk that is secreted by the mammary glands of female mamales to nourish their young. Most often the colostrum is taken from the first 6 to 12 hours of the newborn's life. Colostrum contains the essential nutrients for a young cow to grow, develop and to sustain life. Bovine colostrum (cows) is practically identical to that of human colostrum; however bovine colostrum contains four times the amount of immune factors than that of human colostrum. Colostrum also is rich in growth factors, and immense amount of vitamins,minerals,and an abundance of amino acids, essential and non-essential. It is the fraction of growth factors, that help colostrum release an IgF-1 response, which helps to build lean muscle tissue that has become of interest to bodybuilders. Colostrum is slowly becoming a popular supplement with bodybuilders today, because of its extreme beneficial qualities in health and muscle building capabilities, a natural IgF-1 releaser that can make a difference in your health and muscle building capabilities. (*make sure the colostrum you buy is of the first 6-12 hours of delivery*).

**Deer Antler Extract** – velvet deer antler extract has been used in traditional Chinese medicine for over 2,000 years. It is known for its capabilities for improving everything from overall health and athletic performance. Clinical studies have shown that the IgF-1 found in deer antlers is capable of promoting muscle cell growth, connective tissue, bone, and nerve health. This is because deer antlers are considered as the fastest, natural growing tissue worldwide. This essential element contains more than 70 amino acids that are helpful in building muscle, and fighting the common symptoms of the aging process.

Now a days people are conducting several studies and research works on the positive side of deer antler extract to humans. The deer antler extract for bodybuilding has shown an intense growth effects among athletes and bodybuilders. The ability of IgF-1 can stimulate the natural growth of muscles twice as powerful than any other supplements. Deer antler extract can help you build muscle faster, improve you recovery response, and benefit your overall health. This supplement you can definitely feel working the first week of use, as I can attest to that myself. It just gets better week after week. Just make sure when buying you buy from a reliable source, as there are many counterfiters out there. *A good one is from "Maxlife Direct, Now, and Nutronicslabs.com", you won't be disappointed !*

**Tongkat Ali** – this product comes from the island of Sumatra and is rapidly becoming depleted because of its capabilities in producing high amounts of testosterone. You might want to consider this herbal product as a natural aphrodisiac, in which it is also primarily used as such in Sumatra, and in the rest of the world. This product is primarily used as an aphrodisiac, and as a treatment for erectile dysfunction in men. The bodybuilding community caught on about this herbal and realized that it increases testosterone quite significantly. Tongkat Ali raises levels of testosterone four times the amount of what the body produces normally. But thats not all it does, it also inhibits *sex hormone binding globumin* (SHBG) thus assuring for more available free testosterone in the blood stream. It is this free testosterone that exerts its affect, not total testosterone in the blood stream, but it's the free(available) testosterone that makes muscles grow. Tongkat can boost your testosterone back up to more youthful levels, increasing your capability to increase more muscle mass. *Make sure when purchasing you get the Sumatran brand 200:1 extract and not the Indonisian one.*

**Bulbine Natalensis Extract** – A native herb from South Africa that may in small dosages substantially increase testosterone quickly, while at the same time reduce estrogen levels by 35%. This herb has recently been receiving a lot of attention from the press for its libido/testosterone boosting abilities. Bulbine, seems to also be the only herbal extract that can raise testosterone and lower estrogen at the same time. *When taking Bulbine, make sure to cycle it, 2 weeks on, 1 week off, and you also do not need large dosages, only a small amount is needed for its affects, more is not necessarily better when it comes to Bulbine. You also have to make sure when buying this extract, it* *is freeze dried.*

**Suma Root extract** – a product of South America that has been used in Brazil as an aphrodisiac, a general tonic, and just a bout what ails the human body. Suma root is known for its content of (beta-ecdysterone) that has anabolic properties. Due to its anabolic action, suma root is now being used as a natural anabolic to build muscle and help treat chronic fatigue syndrome. Researched heavily by Russian scientists, it was known to contain 19 different amino acids, a large number of electrolytes, trace minerals, vitamins, and pantothenic acid (B5). It also contains a high amount of germanium that accounts for its ability as an oxygenator, and high source of iron content that may account for its traditional uses for anemia. The root also contains phyto chemicals that include saponins, pfaffic acid, glycosides, and nortriterpines. Suma was once called the "Russian Secret" because it was taken at one time by the Russian Athletes during the Olympic Games.

Suma's main anabolic action can be attributed to its high content of beta-ecdysterone and 3 novel ecdysteroid glycosides. Being a rich source of beta-edysterone that is the subject of a Japanese patent that was filed for a US patent in 1998 for a propriety extract of Suma (which extracted the ecdysterone and beta ecdysterone. These researchers claimed through various in vitro and vivo studies that compound maintained health and had other various health benefits as an overall tonic. Look for the highest standardized extract for beta-ecdysterones when buying Suma root.

**Personal note:** *I can honestly say that when you try this extract, providing you get a high standardization, you will appreciate the effects of it.*

**Secretagogue GH-Releaser** – *sold by MHP*, this GH enhancer works in helping the body produce more available growth hormone. Very popular among the anti-aging enthusiants, for its anti-aging affects. This product is good for athletes and bodybuilders that are over 40 years old, as their Gh production is dwindling downwards. A very effective product that you can actually feel working within weeks.

**HGH Up** – *sold by "Applied Nutriceuticals"*, this another GH enhancing product that helps you to produce more GH, also an affective product that works equally well as the Secretagogue. Basically all have similar formula's and ingredients in so many of these GH Enhancers sold today. I'm just listing the ones that in my opinion work very well that I have tried myself.

**Prime** – **by USP Labs**, Prime is a herbal formula that sells very well for USP Labs that is sort a natural anabolic/adaptogen. Helps the body to promote thickness, size, and physical strength.

**Powerful** – **by USP Labs**, this is a very potent GH releaser that sells extremely well, and is usually sold out ! Its main herb is the extract of "Mucuna Prureins" Velvet Bean, which has been the subject of multiple studies on growth hormone. Powerful has one of the strongest extractions of velvet bean on the market today for its L-dopa content, among GH enhancers sold today. You will literally feel it working within days, especially if your 40 years and older. Powerful also has another herbal compound from the herb Chlorophytum Boriviianum, that has specific Triterpene steroidal saponins and sapogonegins that boost the already power effect from the velvet bean extract, L-dopa. The formula sold today is a much stronger one than what was sold last year. Reviews have been solid for this amazing product.

**Pink Magic** – *sold by USP Labs*, another fine product from USP Labs that is also very popular among the bodybuilders and gym enthsuiants. Pink magic is a herbal formula that consists of three powerful herbs in their own right, but when grouped together, you have a powerful combination with results that speak for itself. Pink Magic is kind of a testosterone booster with an adaptogenic affect that helps prevent catabolism within muscle tissue and provides more for an anabolic environment thats favorable for muscle growth.

**Test Powder** – sold by USP labs, this is one of USP Labs newer products that just was recently introduced on the market, and I must say that the ingredients really interested me, that I am looking forward in trying it myself ! The ingedients consist of an amino acid /herbal formula of "Mucuna Prureins" extract of 200mgs and D-Aspartic Acid, Trimethylglycine,Carnitine Tartrate, and several other ingredients as well, to me looks very promising as a well developed formula by a company that takes geat pride in producing great products, and actually all of their products are great. Some of them have won supplement of the year. But based on USPLabs reputation i'm going to give this a try myself.

**SuperCissus-RX** - yep you guess it ! Another USP Lab product is one of my favorites that I personally always use on a consistent level. Cissus is a herb from India that has amazing anabolic properties for strengthening tendons, and ligaments. It has won supplement of the year for that reason. This patent pending product has quickly established itself among customers and industry insiders alike. It has won numerous awards as the #1 joint product of the year for 2008 and 2009. They key ingredient is "Cissus Quandrangularis" that has been supported by centuries of use in Ayuredic Traditional Medicine in India, it has also been the subject of numerous clinical studies. Great to use for nagging joint related problems and trouble area's of the body from stress induced bodybuilding. Its anabolic affect for muscle building properties can be compared to the steroid "D-Ball" Dianabol. With that,enough said ! This is one product that you shouldn't be without, trust me on this one,especially this one !

**HumanoGrowth** – *from Labrada Nutrition*, Humanogrowth is a cutting edge embryonic peptide matrix (standardized chicken embryo extract) developed in Eastern Europe, designed to help the body support testosterone production and decrease recovery time. Humanogrowth contains naturally occurring growth factors that have a unique bio-stimulating properties; like IGF-1, IGF-2, FGF- Fibroblast growth factors, NGF-Nerve growth factors, EGF- Embryo growth factors, and CTGF -Connective tissue growth factors. HumanoGrowth is not your ordinary testosterone-booster, but a highly developed cutting edge supplement that is geared to help your body produce growth promoting fractions that stimulate muscle tissue growth and increase your recovery time for complete recuperation. This a supplement that you stay on and the results are kind of accumilative. Again a good product for muscle building.

**Tribulus Terrestris Extract** – Bulgarian tribulus is a quality testosterone booster that has been made very popular quickly by the Bulgarian Olympic Weightlifting team years ago, and to which is still very popular today. Tribulus must be bought in a high quality extract standardized for its steroidal saponins, the percentage of saponins should be 40% or higher if you are going to see results. Tribulus has a *unique ability in increasing levels of (LH) leutenizing hormone which in turn spurs significant increases in the levels of testosterone.* In addition to its testosterone boosting affect, There were two solid tribulus studies suggesting that it was also found to be a nitric oxide stimulator. Nitric oxide can significantly impact muscle contractility and nutrient metabolism. Also in the findings of the two studies were that the nitric oxide release from tribulus would explain the nitric oxide release from the nerve endings which stimulates the Corpus Cavernosum ( tissue responsible for erections) and increases in blood flow. Tribulus is also found in many of the testosterone boosting formula's on the market today, because it works!

**Androtest** – rated as the industries protodioscin content leader, androtest is another herbal formula that has powerful testosterone boosting capabilities to help build muscle. The formula consists of two of the most natural potent testosterone producing herbs, Tribulus is one of the ingredients in androtest that is standardized to 40% to 48% protodioscin, and Tongkat Ali being the other powerful active ingredient standardized for its quassinoid content. Androtest impressively, in one clinical study increased levels of DHEA by 47%, SHBG decreased by 66% and the free available testosterone index escalated by 73%. This new generation of protodioscin-rich tribulus, and Tongkat Ali represent what may be the single most
potent and natural testosterone producing supplement on the market today. Look for androtest on the Prosource.net site on the internet.

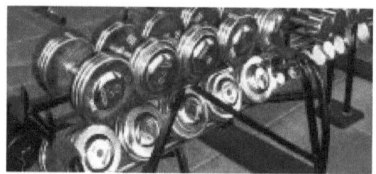

## Chapter 16
## <u>HOW TO BEST USE</u>
## <u>PRE-WORKOUT/POST-WORKOUT SUPPLEMENTS</u>

With so many different choices of what supplement to use for your pre-workouts and post workouts, we often get confused on all the available supplements to choose from. Every manufacturer claims that their product is better than their competitions. Who are you suppose to believe ? Well, some may say that if you're eating a substantial diet and you're getting all the required nutrients, you shouldn't really need to be spending your money on extra supplements, when you can get the same results from foods. But contrary to what they may say, pre-workout supplements are necessary for optimal performance during your training routine.

With the cutting edge technology in sports nutrition, sports manufacture's have come along way in this field, and it is kind of difficult getting certain ingredients that are in supplements from the foods we eat. Currently the best pe-workout supplements on the market contain the necessary ingredients such as *nitric oxide, amino acids, caffeine, creating, beta-alaline, citrulline, AAKG, etc.*, just to name a few. Pre-workout supplements are specifically designed for just that purpose, pre-workouts! And certain ingredients that are available today, is just too impossible to get from certain foods, plus you would have to consume probably large amounts of it to get the same effect as if would take it in 3-to-4 pills.

They are tailored made for a specific biological function, and that is to provide you with energy, endurance, pump, and muscular growth. There has been a surge of new studies and information about the positive effects of pre-workout supplementation. With that in mind it's no wonder that supplement manufacture's have been taking advantage of this by producing huge amounts of pre-workout supplements. The next time you are in a GNC, take a look around their shelves and see that there is such a wide array of pre-workout supplements. Back in the 70's when I started training we didn't have available from the amount that you have to choose from, and as a matter of fact, we didn't have any period!

I would always say to myself, "if they would only make something like a pre-workout supplement that will give you a big boost in your training"
back then, we had to rely on oatmeal, extra B vitamins, and banana's for a extra boost of energy.

I knew at that time that some kind of pre-workout supplementation was important for training and muscle growth. Now there are so many to choose from that it would make one's head spin, and most of the choices you choose, would be trial and error, till you found one that really worked. Let's face it, it really is a big market with so many people taken part in fitness programs and diets, that now its all about looking buff and muscular. There are also many bogus pre-workout supplements that really don't do diddly and the ingredients are not what they claim to be. It really is that type of a market out there, every manufacture jumps on the band wagon of riches ripping us off of our hard earned money.

I will show you what the decent pre-workout supplements are and what brands are reputable to buy. Today we have a myraid of different combinations of ingredients, but they all tend to have the same basic ingredient combinations, just in different dosages. I can't say that they all work, cause I haven't tried all of them, but I can say what works on the one's that I did try, and some of them worked better than they advertised. <u>Your basic pre-workout supplements consists of the following ingredients:</u>

- **creating**
- **whey protein**
- **carbohydrates (dextrose & maltodextrin)**
- **flavoring**

This is a basic pre-workout formula, and you want to know something ? It works ! I can tell you now, that by taking a pre-workout supplement consisting of the above ingredients of whey, creatine, and carbs will greatly improve blood flow and will help provide your body with a constant supply of amino acids and glucose while working out. This in turn will help prevent muscle tissue break down during your workouts, suppress cortisol build-up, and improve energy.

Again we are faced with the dilemma, which one is the best one ? Well, there really isn't just one best pre-workout supplement out there, there's many that work very well, it's a simple matter of knowing the basics of what your body needs nutritionally, as far as whats needed for a pre-workout requirement based on the task at hand. For one we are lifting weights, which puts a stress demand on the muscles and two, we know now what muscles need for growth, and three, a nutrient to sustain our exercise capacity endurance wise. This is how I go about in choosing a pre-workout supplement for my particular needs.

Always look at the ingredients and judge for yourself asking, does this particular supplement meet my physical and biological demand. Are the ingredients enough for me to provide energy,stamina, and growth ?
That is how I determine my pre-workout supplement. I also consider the manufacturer's reputation and quality of their products. It's going to be a matter of trial and error as well, on what worked well for you. But I will list some supplements that I have tried myself, that do work pretty well, and some that are worth mentioning as well.

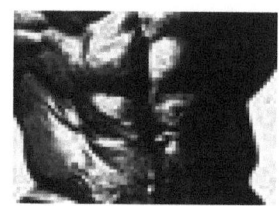

## CHAPTER 17
## PRE-WORKOUT SUPPLEMENTS

**1.     USP Labs – (Jack3dMicro)** -A company that always produces top of the line quality and products that deliver. Jack3dMicro is a new pre-workout formula of the previous Jack3d, has some very interesting ingredients that I'm kind of excited about and looking forward in trying myself, I'm a big follower of the USP labs line for their great formulated products that have never failed. This one looks like a keeper!

**2.     USP Labs – (Jack3d)** -Excellent formula that you can feel working right from the first serving. (great feedback from this product)

**3.     MHP's (NO-BOMB)** -This is another quality company that gets good reviews from their product line. NO-BOMB is a revolutionary nitric oxide booster that will give you incredible muscle pumps, sustained energy and strength. The formulation of this product is a sound one with ingredients you can feel working.

**4.     MHP – (TRAC Extreme)** – A powerful formula that really boosts the nitric oxide level to where you can get awesome muscle pumps and energy that keeps you going without feeling that wired jittery feeling. Trac is a product that works very well ! Loaded with nutrients making this a powerfull pe-workout formula.

**5.     Gaspari Nutrition -(Super Pump Max)** –A pre-workout supplement that produces skin tearing pumps, great reviews ! Packed with branched amino acids,nitric oxide boosters, electrolytes,creatine, and nutritionalco-factors. The Gaspari line is also another reputable company that poduces quality products.

6.	**BPI-Sports (1.M.R.)** -BPI Sports supplement line is relatively new product line has been getting some great reviews lately. Excellent company with products that deliver results. I have personally tried some of them with great satisfaction. Provides the user with a sustained amount of energy and pumps without that jittery feeling which most pre-workout supplements give.

7.	**Gaspari Nutrition -(Vasotropin)** -Advertised as the "Ultimate Pump Solution" this formula utilizes some high-tech nutritional ingredients that promises top deliver sustained energy levels with unbelievable pumps. Expensive product, but the Gaspari line of supplements are backed by research and has never produced a non-quality product.

8.	**Millennium Sports Technologies – (Cordygen 5)** - A patented formula that incorporates a blend of 5 strains and 4 species of the cordyceps mushroom extract 100% USDA certified organic and highly concentrated in a time-released formula. Cordyceps helps you maximize oxygen utilization for sustained levels of endurance and muscular strength. Cordygen 5 is used by the top athletes around the world for its ability in increasing oxygen utilization, strength, endurance, and sustained energy levels. (One of my personal favorites).

9.	**Millennium Sports Technologies – (Ultra Cordygen Vo2)** Aame as above but new and improved, super potent ! Maximizes oxygen utilization, decreases oxygen debt,maximizes endurance,increases Vo2 max,and increases ATP production.

10.	**BSN – (Hyper FX)** A very good company that caters to bodybuilding supplements. Hyper FX is a good pre-workout supplement that is packed with nutrition.

11.	**CytoSports – (CytoMax)** This is an exercise and recovery drink formulated with an advanced complex carbohydrate, electrolyte performance and recovery drink. CytoMax ensures you to stay positively hydrated, steady energy levels,and helps you to minize post exercise muscle soreness. Cytomax also helps to buffer lactic-acid production in muscle tissue allowing you to train longer and recovery quickly. Great pre-workout supplement !

12.	**Athletic Edge Nutrition -(IntraXcell)** This a beta-alanine formula that's been backed by major university, peer reviewed studies performed on humans, not the typical cell or rat studies upon many other manufactures generally base claims on. Beta-Alanine has been shown to boost muscular strength, muscular anaerobic endurance,increase aerobic endurance,and increase exercise capacity so you could train harder and longer.

13.	**Metabolic Nutrition – (C.G.P.)** Creatine glycerol phosphate, a new patented creating formula that is able to accelerate absorption in the G.I. Tract via a specialized pathway
that eliminates all the negative side effects associated with most creatine products. C.G.P. Serves as its own high energy phosphate and electrolyte reservoir contributing to the production of ATP, delaying fatigue,increasing strength, and magnifying endurance.

**14.    Applied Nutraceuticals – (Lit-Up)** This product utilizes the most cutting edge formulation that yields cumulative results in that it increases energy levels, testosterone, and functions as an anticatabolic, suppressing cortisol and increases the mind to muscle connection.

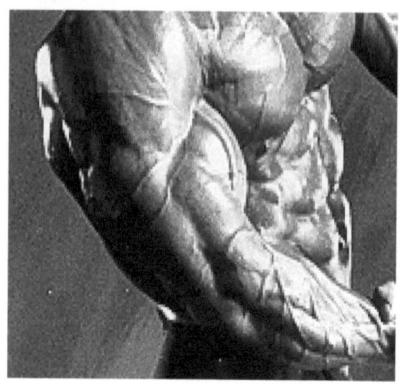

## CHAPTER 18
## Post-Workout Supplements

Your post-workout nutrition is probably your most important part of your day regarding muscular growth, and so, here we are again in choosing the best possible post-workout supplementation for our muscle building purposes. As with pre-workout supplements, it is the same dilemma in choosing the best supplement for post workouts. You also learned earlier in previous chapters on the importance of nutrient timing and what we need nutritionally, how much is needed ? And of what we need to satisfy our post workout recovery process.

But, what we are looking for in terms of supplementation is a good protein powder or meal replacement powder that can meet our nutritional requirements that we have established for ourselves for maximum growth. So, your best bet is to choose a high quality protein supplement fortified with vitamins,minerals,enzymes, and essential fats.The whole enchilada !

My ideal post-workout supplement is a **whey hydrolyzed protein powder** that I can mix in with, -flax seed oil,carbohydrate powder(dextrose),10 grams of extra glutamine, colostrum powder, and a vitamin-mineral powder that I buy separately and add in, or I can just avoid all the mix and match, and search for a high quality meal replacement powder that might have all the necessary nutrients in it already. Personally when your at it as long as I have been, and I'm sure this goes the same for the rest of the experienced bodybuilders, is to mix and match my protein with the necessary co-factors (nutrients) that I mentioned before. For me, my post-workout shake or meal is the opportune time for anabolic activity to take place, and so I want to make sure i'm not leaving anything out, **such as:**

## Ultimate Protein Muscle Building Shake

**Protein source should be** of a high quality **whey protein powder** (consider *hydrolysates first and isolates second, and glutamine peptide's.* (for its rapid absorption into the intestines) Add in a scoop of **Egg protein powder** as well. For their high biological value.Making sure you're getting at least 40 to 50 grams of protein in your shake.

**Carbohydrate should be** – Glucose(dextrose) or carbohydrates that generate glucose (maltodextrin). Glucose will help to restore muscle and liver glycogen reserves, which will trigger an insulin response, helping with protein synthesis.

**Essential fatty Acids should be** -Fats that are digested fast, like MCT's(medium chain triglycerides), coconut oil, avocado oil, macadamia oil, lecithin, ALA.

**Creatine powder** – known as one of the greatest muscle-building supplements ever. Include at least 5-10 grams of creating powder to your mix to help with your recovery, and muscle growth process.

**Other great ingredients I like to Add in:**

**Colostrum Powder** – For it's growth promoting factors, IgF-1 & 2,immune enhancing compounds, vitamins, minerals, and fats.

**Enzymes (Papaya/Bromelian)** – To help with better intestinal absorption of nutrients and digestion.

**Glutamine Powder** - (personal choice) As glutamine will help with better intestinal health and muscle induced damage from exercise, and in the recovery process.

**All One /Vitamin & Mineral Powder – a little insurance won't hurt! Or you can add an anti oxidant blend instead.**

**Overview:**
Having the proper supplementation readily available for consumption post-workout, can drastically improve your ability to enhance your muscle growth capabilities. A high quality nutrient dense post-workout supplement **(as in above)** can complement your training in providing you with the macro and micro nutrients so necessary in achieving fast muscular growth.
There are some readily made quality protein shakes available, but they don't compare to my ultimate protein shake ! (I use the ultimate shake only on workout days) and it would be wise of you if you do the same, if your interested in fast muscle growth. However, I will also list some of the better quality protein powders that you may be interested in seeing.

**Post-Workout Protein Shakes**

1.      **Optimum Nutrition's (Platinum Hydro-Builder)** – a very good formula that contains high quality hydrolysates for rapid digestion, and mixes so easily. Contains 30 grams of protein perserving with 5 grams of micronized creatine, and a enzyme complex.

2.      **Optimum Nutrition's (Hydro-Whey)** – contains the same quality hydrolysates and protein per serving except it lacks the added micronized creatine.

3.      **Gaspari Nutrition (Size On)** – a formula thats based on valied clinical research. Contains a hybred Intra workout whey hydrolysate creatine formula with outlast carbohydrate matrix. Designed to promote maximum muscle volume and accelerate protein synthesis. Loaded with amino acids and vitamins and minerals.

4.      **MusceTech (Anabolic Halo Hardcore Series)** – this is a high tech cutting edge formula featuring micro-difuse technology. Contains creating that is loaded with powerful amino acids, vitamins, and minerals with nutritional cofactors.

5.      **Optimum Nutrition (2:1 Recovery)** – this recovery shake contains carbohydrates in a 2:1 ratio perfect for post workout recovery. Hydrolyzed whey protein is the protein source for quick digestion.(this product is great to use as a base when mixing your own post-workout blend).

6.      **MHP – (Dark Matter)** – absorbs faster than whey isolates with a 600% increase in protein synthesis equal to 40 grams of protein. Contains a multi-phase hydro-size creating transport. Dramatically spikes insulin levels with WaxiMax-CG3, and replenishes glycogen and increases cell volume.

7.      **CytoSports -(Muscle Milk)** – a unique protein blend Eva-Pro that contains alpha and beta micellar caseins with a precise mix to stimulate anabolic gowth. Essential fatty acids are added to fortify the blend and creatine factors in optimizing your body's own capability to manufacture optimal levels of creatine.(this is a very good formula)

8.      **CytoSport – (Monster Mass)** a high calorie nutrient dense post-workout shake that has everything you could want in it, quality protein mix,fats,carbs,vitamins,creatine,minerals in a easily digested protein mix of fast and slow proteins. Monster mass helps you create a positive nitrogen balance, the gold standard of
9.      anabolic potential. Each serving contains 50 grams of protein.

10.     **Champion Nutrition – (Ultra-Met)** is a meal-replacement protein shake made by a reputable company thats been around a while that specializes in sports supplements. Ultra-Met can be used as a breakfast meal, or dinner replacement. Ultra-met also provides 42 grams of nitrogen rich protein, 24 grams of carbohydrates, and 27 vitamins and minerals to support your metabolism.

11.     **Met-Rx (Colossal Meal Re-Placement Bars)** - this is a great way to add extra calories and protein in between hours to fortify your post-workout recovery period for faster growth.

<u>Overview:</u> There are so many brands and formula's to choose from that will make your head spin. The brands of post-workout supplements that I listed is to give you a head start in trying and experimenting with. You will be able to see what works best for you. But, as I mentioned earlier, you can't go wrong with using a
**<u>simple shake made up of:</u>**

➤ **proteins**
➤ **carbohydrates**
➤ **creatine**

You can use this as a starting base point and add slowly certain blends of nutrients and co-factors to create more of a potent recovery muscle building shake.

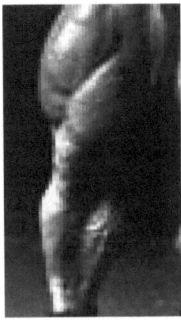

## CHAPTER 19
## <u>BOOSTING YOUR HORMONES FOR MAXIMUM MUSCLE DEVELOPMENT THROUGH DIET & EXERCISES</u>

There are several ways that we can increase our own levels of testosterone and growth hormone, through natural means without resorting to steroids.

One way is by employing certain exercise movements, and the best exercises are compound movements using multiple muscle groups. Examples of this would be squats, bench press, rowing, dead lifts, pull ups, and power cleans.

There are also a couple of things to keep in mind –**<u>Focus on lower body exercises like squats,</u>** that can provide a healthy flow of these powerful hormones in a way the upper lifts won't.

**<u>Focus on power</u>** –making sure that you are focusing on power when you are trying to add size to your frame. Mix up also your sets and reps to cover both the high and low rep counts. But be sure to add power sets in there with lower reps of 3-5 with higher weight added to it. Try at least one to two times a week for a max lift in bench press, dead lifts, power cleans, or high pulls. **<u>Here are four power exercises that will boost your testosterone and GH levels: and add some serious muscle mass.</u>**

1.      **<u>Deadlifts</u>** – This exercise is a must that needs to be in your workout program if you want to add size fast, and build strength.(keep the bar close to your body and focus lifting with your legs, get low and don't let your knees, chest, or face lean forward beyond your toes as your lifting the bar up. Keeping the back straight.

2.      **<u>Power Squats</u>** – Will help you increase your over all size by naturally boosting your  testosterone and Gh much like deadlifts can. When performing power squats make sure no part of your body leans forward past your toes, keep your eyes focused on

looking up at your eye level position from your starting point as you begin squatting down making sure that your buttocks touch your ankles on the down ward part of the movement.

3.    **Power Cleans** – this is considered an Olympic lift that will add size, power and strength to your over all body, and may be the best over all exercise that one never adds to their program. A great hormone booster because of it being an explosive movement. To perform this movement, begin by crouching over the Olympic bar hand grip should be a bout shoulder level, with knees bent slightly and your back more or less parallel to the floor. As you pull the weight past your knees, straighten your body and pull it up to your shoulder position as if you were going to perform a military press. (for those that are not sure how to perform this movement, you tube has excellent video's on this and many other Olympic movements).

4.    **Barbell Bench Press** – when done in the power lifting method, you are doing 1 rep maximum for your greatest amount of weight that you can handle. Trying to complete about 3-5 sets of each. Finish off with medium to light weight on the bar and perform as many reps as you can, then strip off some more weight and perform the max reps as you can do with minimum rest, that is the key for hormonal stimulation.

By knowing how to increase testosterone through certain exercises, we can have the added advantage of manipulating our hormones to build muscle tissue. By performing compound movements with brief high intensity sessions, your body responds by providing short spurts of hormone release, be it testosterone or GH. Heavy weight with 4-6 reps and high intensity sessions are the best in boosting testosterone. Now endurance training on the other hand has a different hormonal effect. It leads to increased "cortisol levels" and low testosterone levels, and that we do not want as cortisol is a catabolic hormone. So, training for long extended periods is detrimental to your testosterone and Gh levels. Workouts should last no more than 45 minutes to an hour at most. Your natural levels of testosterone will peak at 45 minutes into an intense weight training workout. You really do not need to train for longer periods than that, if you workout hard, you will get the results you looking for.

Your diet also plays an important role in boosting your testosterone levels. An extremely low carb and low fat diet will actually decrease your testosterone. Keep healthy carbs and essential fats in your diet, and eat plenty of quality protein.

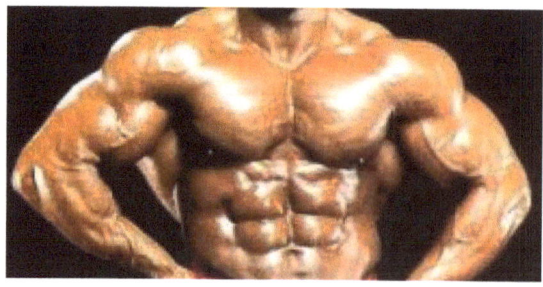

**CHAPTER 20**

# BOOSTING YOUR TESTOSTERONE THROUGH DIET

Add healthy monounsaturated fats like olive oil to your daily diet to help get your daily requirements of up to 35% to 50%, which boosts testosterone. Research by Volek et al. Included in their findings that monounsaturated fats and saturated fat dramatically raised testosterone levels by 62% and 59% respectively. <u>Monounsaturated fats like olive oil, canola oil, nuts, peanut butter, and avocados.</u> Moreover foods high in healthy omega 3 fatty acids would be a great source of testosterone raising fats. <u>With the best source of omega 3 being fatty fish like herring, mackerel, sardines, tuna, and salmon.</u> Omega 3's are also found in plant foods walnuts, pumpkin seeds,flax seeds,and flax seed oil. By keeping your consumption of monounsaturated oils and omega 3's up around 35% to 50%, which is the amount research shows to be optimal for raising your testosterone levels. In addition to healthy fats and Omega 3's for increasing testosterone levels, meat and diary products also are "key" ingredients in any diet based on raising your testosterone levels. The foods listed below are testosterone boosting foods:

- **Meats** –A great source of protein, fats, minerals(zinc & iron), and vitamins. Make sure your cuts of meat are of lean variety.

- **Eggs** – Consists of quality bio-available protein, fats,vitamins, and minerals. Studies also show that the cholesterol found in eggs is not harmful. Eggs are rich in Lecithen and Lecithen is a natural emulsifier. Try and make sure you get in 3 to 4 eggs in your daily diet. Can make a big difference in your muscle building development.

- **Oysters** - A great source of testosterone boosting minerals, especially "zinc" which is required in the metabolism of testosterone. Consuming oysters(raw) at least once a week, is known to make a huge difference in testosterone stimulation.

- **Nuts** –Almonds, cashews, walnuts, peanuts, are some very essential foods in boosting testosterone levels. Also a great nutritious snack in between meals.

- **Beans** – Packed with proteins and zinc are also known to be great testosterone enhancers. Which include soy beans, chick peas, black beans, and kidney beans. They are also low in fat and high in fiber. Ensure that you include a variety of beans in your diet.

- **Dairy** -Get your glass of milk daily, whether it be from skimmed or low fat milk, also include with that yogurt and cottage cheese.

- **Fruits** – There are specific fruits that contain necessary ingredients that are vital in testosterone production, and they include bananas, figs, avocados, and different types of berries. By making a nutritious fruit smoothie with skimmed milk, you will enjoy a power house drink that will give you all the energy and testosterone boosting nutrients.

As you can see there are plenty of foods that can help you in boosting your testosterone levels naturally. You now have a basic blue-print that you can follow with all the necessary ingredients and information in designing a diet that will suit your needs in muscle development.

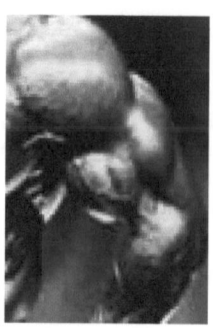

## CHAPTER 21
## TESTOSTERONE & GROWTH HORMONE BOOSTING SUPPLEMENTS

✦ **Tongkat Ali (Eurycoma Longifolia)** - A powerful testosterone boosting herb native to the island of Sumatra, that has been used for many years as an aphrodisiac to help in sexual dysfunction. Tongkat has been shown to increase testosterone levels 4 times higher than normal. Was once made popular on T.V. By Dr.Oz, which helped it increase its popularity. It didn't hurt also that Dr. Oz stated that tongkat just may well be nature's most powerful aphrodisiac. Tongkat Ali's effect on testosterone production was also caught on by the bodybuilding community. A powerful product that should be in every weightlifters shelf for the ultimate stimulation of testosterone for those looking for a strong natural testosterone-booster. Make sure it is of the Sumatran brand and is in a 200:1 extract form. Bodybuilders typically take about 400 to 800 mgs of this herb, but for those just trying it out for the first time I would suggest half of that amount. Make sure also that when taking Tongkat Ali,to cycle it for 4 weeks and 2 weeks off.

✦ **Tribulus Terristris** – A high standardized extract(40% or higher) of tribulus terristris can help you build muscle and increase your sexual performance. Tribulus stimulates testosterone in an indirect way by stimulating a hormone called Luetenizing Hormone in the pituitary gland. Which later is converted in the leydig cells of the scrotum into testosterone. Scientists at the Chemical Pharmaceutical Research Institute in Sofia, Bulgaria demonstrate that supplementation with tribulus terristris increased testosterone production by 30%. For an even greater effect in boosting testosterone, you can combine tribulus with tongkat ali. Tribulus must be cycled on and off for greater effects, 4 weeks on and 2 weeks off.

✦ **Powerful (USP Labs)** –This is a great GH supplement that generally sells out due to its great affect on GH. Powerful contains the herb Mucuna Prureins for its high L-dopa content that has been known to be a great GH stimulator.

✦ **Deer Antler Velvet** – (Nutronics Labs) Nutronic labs sells the strongest formula of deer antler on the market today. This product was made very popular by professional fottball players and the major league baseball players for its potent IgF-1 release (insulin-growth-factor-1). Deer antler's have been used for thousands of years by the Chinese for its health rejuvenating affect on the body. This supplement will definitely make a big difference in your muscle development quickly, its that potent ! Combined with a good testosterone boosting diet and high protein shakes, you'll be on your way to looking as muscular as you wish to be.

⅄ **Bulbine Natalensis** – this powerful testosterone boosting herb is one of the only herbs to raise testosterone while at the same time lowering estrogen levels by 35%. A native to South Africa, bulbine is starting to make its way into the bodybuilding stage. Not much is needed in order to get a testosterone boost, but if taken too much, you then risk the chance of decreasing your testosterone. As with all herbal testosterone boosting supplements, Bulbine should be cycled on for 4 weeks and off for 2 weeks. (remember, taking more of this herb does not result in more of a testosterone increase, with this herb, less is better).

⅄ **MuscleMeds – (Methyl-Arimatest)** a unique formula in that it functions as a testosterone booster and an anti-aromatase inhibitor keeping testosterone from metabolizing into estrogen. A cutting edge supplement from an excellent company that delivers with results you can see and feel.

Testosterone boosting supplements and GH enhancers can make a big difference in the rate of which you can build quality muscle. Together, along with a good training program and a carefully thought out diet plan, there is no limit and amount of muscle growth that you can obtain.

In closing, I would like to add that just because we have approached middle age, it does not mean that we have to settle for mediocrity. I have made available to you in the most simple way of to build muscle in your advanced year's. Like they often say, it's never too late to begin training at any age. Never let anyone ever tell you that you're too old to do anything in life, as they don't call the "Golden Years of You're Life" golden for no reason at all,

Its golden because you are at a prime time of you're life. So, let's start training and build yourself a body that you can be proud of. I wish you the best of health and physical fitness, for many years to come. Good luck to You!